FOREWORD

If out of the abundance of the heart the mouth speaketh and writeth then Rev. Oden surely has a noble soul.

He has made an enduring contribution to the cause of Christianity in particular and justice and freedom in general.

He renews our conviction in the rightness of our cause by reviving our awareness of eternal truths.

He has said so much which so desparately needed to be said with more wisdom and insight and just plain goodness than any book I have ever read on the subject.

He has made us even prouder that we have been the roots of a movement which we are deeply convicted serves both God and country.

May God bless Rev. Oden as richly as he has blessed us with this God guided book.

Maureen Salaman
Co-editor "The Choice" magazine

INTERNATIONAL ASSOCIATION OF
CANCER VICTIMS and FRIENDS, INC.
TWIN CITIES CHAPTER
151 Silver Lake Rd. Suite 7
St. Paul, Minnesota 55112

THANK GOD
I HAVE CANCER!

REV. CLIFFORD ODEN

FREEDOM of CHOICE PUBLISHERS INC.

LOS ALTOS, CALIFORNIA

This book is written for religious and educational purposes only.
It is not to be used commercially to promote the sale of any product
mentioned herein or to solicit business for any organization
mentioned herein.

Copyright © 1976 by Clifford E. Oden

All rights reserved. No portion of this book may
be reproduced without written permission from the
publisher except by a reviewer who may quote brief
passages in connection with a review.

Library of Congress Cataloging in Publication Data

Oden, Clifford E
   Thank God I have cancer!
   1. Cancer—Personal narratives. 2. Faith-cure—
Personal narratives. 3. Oden, Clifford E. I. Title.
RC263.03   616.9'94'06520924 [B]   76-9824
ISBN 0-87000-262-3

This volume is dedicated to
LOUISE
my faithful companion for thirty-six years,
without whose prayers the truths contained herein
might never have been discovered,
and without whose help and encouragement
this work could not have been produced.

Table of Contents

PREFACE ....
1. GOD WANTS US TO BE WELL ....
2. FOOD IS THE PRIMARY SOURCE OF HEALTH .
3. MAN IS RESPONSIBLE FOR DISEASE ....
4. NO ONE CAN HEAL YOU BUT YOURSELF .....
5. THE WORLD OPPOSES GOD'S WAY OF HEALING.....................................
6. THE MALIGNANT CELL IS A NORMAL PART OF LIFE ....
7. GOD PROVIDES FOR CANCER CONTROL IN NATURE ....
8. THE MAJORITY OPINION IS OFTEN ATHEISTIC AND WRONG................................
9. IT IS "ILLEGAL" FOR GOD TO RELIEVE CANCER MISERY ....
10. WE CAN COOPERATE WITH GOD ANYWAY ...
11. WE ARE ALL TERMINAL! ....
12. HONEST MEN, MUST SUPPORT FREEDOM OF CHOICE ....
APPENDIX ....

PREFACE

So you think I'm crazy! And I don't blame you. A few years ago I might have thought the same about anyone who was thankful for cancer. But today I can truly say from my heart that I am grateful to the Lord for permitting me to have this much-feared disease. Why? Many persons have benefited from the things I have learned as a cancer victim. A few cancer patients are alive today, several have reduced their suffering, and many are less terrified than before because of information which I learned and shared with them. Of course they could have secured this information many other places, but I happened to be the channel through which God chose to help them. That is why I am grateful. What I at first thought was a disaster has turned out to be a blessing in disguise. Of course this should not have surprised me or anyone else because the Lord has promised us that "all things work together for good to them that love God, to them who are the called according to His purpose" (Rom. 8:28). And this verse explains that God uses all these things (including seeming tragedies) to make His children more like Christ. And so I have learned to be grateful for every experience that God uses to make me more useful in His service. Quite a few of God's people have stated that my experience with malignancy has benefited them by showing how they could better cope with the same disease. This has been a real joy, and so I can sincerely say "Thank you, Lord for permitting me to have cancer!"

HOW IT ALL STARTED

I knew something was terribly wrong by the tone of the doctor's voice on the telephone. He said, "I sure need to see you right away." A few days before he had taken a biopsy from the descending colon, and when I heard the tone of his voice, I suspected the worst. The blood drained from my face and the strength went out of my hands. I could hardly drive my car to his office. His report was what I feared: cancer of the colon! The only hope was an immediate colostomy. No other alternative! The time schedule? Within a week! The prediction? Five years!

I was not afraid of surgery nor opposed to surgery, but I did face a tremendous problem. I did not know for sure that this was God's will in my case. I had read that cancer treatments were highly controversial. I also realized that while surgery often helped the cancer victim, there were other times when it merely spread the disease. Furthermore I had read where several reputable authorities estimated that 20% of surgery in this country was unnecessary!

So my problem was to find God's will for my particular situation. What if I had this troublesome procedure and later learned that God had another plan for me? How terrible! So I turned to prayer. I asked my friends to pray. I immediately sent out hundreds of letters to Christians and preacher friends all over America. Dozens of churches in many states called special prayer meetings for me. Of course this was not unusual. The same has been done for many other persons, but the nature of the prayer was unusual. I was not praying primarily for my life to be spared. There was no immediate danger, for the malignancy did not seem to be that far advanced. I was not praying primarily for a supernatural healing, although I knew that the Lord often did just that. My wife and I and many of the others were asking for something much greater. We were praying that God would enable me to learn something about the cancer mystery that would be a help to other people. That prayer has been answered in a most wonderful way. Thank you, Lord! If I had received an immediate miraculous healing, I would be the only patient to benefit. But the answer was much greater than such a miracle, for it has opened the door to help for many others besides myself.

At this writing, more than seven years later, I still have not had the surgery. Nine different physicians, all of them in good standing and some of them internationally famous, have confirmed that the malignancy does exist, but so far it has been controlled by natural means without surgery, without radiation, without chemotherapy. It is a lifelong battle, but so far the Lord has kept me winning. I am very grateful to Him for that, and also very grateful for what I have been able to share with others.

THE PURPOSE OF THIS BOOK

I wrote this book because I *must* do so. I asked God for wisdom that I might help others. He answered the prayer, and so I must share the information. It is important that the reader understand that the primary purpose of this book is to honor and praise the Lord Jesus Christ. Its purpose is not to give medical advice to any individual. Of course, if any reader can improve his health as a result of what is written here—praise the Lord!

The best thing that could happen to a cancer patient would be to find a physician who understands God's principles of health. When the physician and the patient and the Lord are cooperating and following the same principles, then of course the best possible results can be expected.

This book was written primarily for Christians, those who have trusted Jesus Christ as Lord and Saviour. Its purpose is to strengthen the faith of the believer by showing that wonderful things the Lord has done for us in the realm of nature. When we realize that God had placed disease-fighting mechanisms in our bodies and in our food supply, we want to cry out with the Psalmist "O Lord, how great are thy works!" (Ps. 92:5).

If this book should fall into the hands of a skeptic, an infidel, an unbeliever, of course such a reader will not believe that God is able to place cytotoxic (cancer-fighting) materials in nature, and of course this writer will appear to be a "nut" in the mind of such a reader. But that is just fine! I would prefer that those who have little respect for our Lord would also have little respect for me. That puts me in better company than I deserve! Jesus said, "If the world hate you, ye know that it hated me before it hated you" (John 15:18).

THE PRINCIPLES I HAVE LEARNED

The Lord has answered my prayer by enabling me to learn some tremendously vital principles about life and health and healing. They are not new, for there is a vast amount of literature on the subject in many languages. Yet these principles are still hidden from the majority because they are not promoted by the most powerful institutions in our society. In fact, those in power often oppose these principles for reasons that will become apparent later.

At the age of fifty I was an average middleclass American with two college degrees and many credit hours beyond—a pastor, teacher, writer, fairly well informed on a wide variety of subjects. But I knew nothing about health; I trusted that to the "experts." And I never would have learned anything about health if I had not been driven to prayer by my cancer experience. I never would have learned anything about health from the usually recognized sources of learning because health is life, and life is from God, and the Scripture says that "the world by wisdom knew not God" (1 Cor. 1:21). God had to make me willing to learn from sources generally considered unorthodox. I had to learn that the majority is not usually right, that the prevailing philosophy of healing is not necessarily correct just because it is promoted by powerful organizations. I had to learn that "God hath chosen the foolish things of the world to confound the wise" (1 Cor. 1:27).

Reader, you will never learn the greatest principles of life and health from the "official" teachings of our society. If you learn from God, you will have to be willing to learn from sources that are "unorthodox" and even despised by those in worldly power (1 Cor. 1:28).

I do not know how these principles may apply

to your own individual needs. But I do hope that when your eyes are opened, as mine were, you will have a deeper appreciation of the goodness of God as revealed in nature.

I am listing here the great lessons God has enabled me to learn as a result of my experience. I wish to share them with you. Each will be discussed in separate sections following.

"In every thing give thanks"
(1 Thessalonians 5:18)

I can thank God even for cancer, because it led me to understand this very encouraging truth—

PRINCIPLE NO. 1: GOD WANTS US TO BE WELL

It is amazing how many Christians are confused about physical health. Many have the idea that God is only concerned with our spiritual welfare and not our physical welfare. But the Apostle Paul prayed that our "spirit and soul and body" be preserved (1 Thess. 5:23). God created man; He is concerned for the welfare of the whole person, including the body. Jesus healed sick bodies as well as sick souls. John prayed that his friend Gaius might have physical health as well as spiritual health (3 John 2).

DON'T BLAME GOD FOR SICKNESS

Some even imagine that God is generally responsible for our sickness. I have heard many a mother complain, "I guess it just isn't God's will for my children to have good health." I can take one look at the child's eating and health habits and a major reason for the poor health becomes obvious. Mother may be destroying her child and blaming it on God!

God wants you well, not sick. Now I realize that this is a broad generalization, and of course there may be exceptions. God *permits* sickness; He may even use sickness as a blessing in disguise—He did in my case (Rom. 8:28). But those who wish to blame God for the generally poor health of believers will have to search the Scriptures thoroughly for some mighty skimpy bits of evidence. Everywhere we look in the Word of God or in nature, we see abundant evidence that God generally promotes health, not disease. Healing is built into nature. Plants, animals, and human beings normally heal automatically.

It has been pointed out by others that the human brain is similar to a vast computer, much more complex than any man-made computer. In case of illness or injury, the brain tells every organ in the body just what to do to bring about the needed repair. The thrilling fact about this is that our computer-brain is programmed before birth to do all this! Now just who programmed it? God did! God did not program the brain to destroy the body, but to preserve and repair the body! So God planned health. He did not plan disease!

GOD'S LAWS OF HEALTH ARE UNIVERSAL

We are not referring to *law* in a legal sense, as a judicial enactment. We refer to law in the scientific sense, as an unvarying principle. We speak of certain natural laws such as gravity. When we call this a law, we mean a universal principle that always holds true without respect to any person or time or place. If a man falls from a great height, gravity will bring him to his death regardless of whether he is Christian or pagan. The law is not personal, but universal!

Likewise, God's laws of health are not personal, but universal. Some of God's best known laws of health are these: proper food, proper exercise, a clean physical environment free of pollution, and a pleasant emotional environment free of stress. These principles promote health; violate these principles and disease results, without regard to the individual. There are millions of pagans in the land of Hunza, a small Asiatic kingdom, and other lands who are in spiritual darkness. Yet they obey God's physical laws of health. They live entirely on natural foods, and they have no diabetes, no cancer, no arthritis, and no heart attacks. Here in "civilized" America there are multitudes of spiritual Christians whose physical diet consists entirely of the artificial man-made foods that our economy dictates we must eat. And they are sick. They die before their time with the very diseases that the "primitive" societies do not have. So you see, God's laws of physical health work regardless of the moral or spiritual condition of the individual. And being universal, they work whether we realize it or not.

GOD WANTS A CLEAN TEMPLE

If you are a true believer in the Lord Jesus Christ, then God's Spirit dwells within you. Your body is the temple of the Holy Spirit (1 Cor. 6:19), and God has done His part to keep this temple healthy. He has programmed your body for health. He has established simple laws or principles which will promote health if we observe them. The rest is up to us. Will we appreciate what He has done? Are we willing to learn the principles of health? Will we cooperate with these principles? If we do, the God-hating world around us may think us strange. But if we violate the principles He has established, we show contempt for the wisdom of God and bring about the premature collapse of our own physical being.

This suggests a most searching question. How great is our guilt if we destroy our own health after God has done so much to promote that health? *Is it not a sin to be sick if we could be well?* I learned this principle too late, but I thank God I finally learned it, even though it took cancer to drive me to this realization. Yet I can still help others to realize that God wants us to be well!

"In every thing give thanks"
(1 Thessalonians 5:18)

I can thank God for cancer, because it led me to appreciate this basic and vital principle—

PRINCIPLE NO. 2: FOOD IS THE PRIMARY SOURCE OF HEALTH

The prevailing view of food in our society reveals an abysmal degree of ignorance. Food in the stomach is thought to be like fuel in a furnace. It supposedly makes little difference what kind of fuel is thrown in the furnace; it will all burn. But the fuel aspect of food is the least vital of its functions. The primary function of food is to supply the building blocks from which the body is constructed and repaired. Therefore it makes a vital difference that we eat. This fact may be obscured by commercial food processors, but it is an elementary principle of biochemistry and thoroughly supported by the Word of God.

THE BIBLE EMPHASIS ON FOOD

I would like to make one point very clear. I am an old-fashioned Baptist preacher with strong orthodox and conservative inclinations. I believe in stressing the same basic Bible principles that our spiritual forefathers have stressed for centuries—such as the sin of man, the deity of Christ, His blood atonement, bodily resurrection, and salvation by grace. I believe these are the most important things, and I do not believe that we should use the Bible primarily to promote some secondary doctrine. This book does deal with nutrition, which is God's natural way of health. I try to write and preach and teach on *every* Biblical subject that can glorify God and benefit man, including health. But I have written and spoken on the great Bible themes at least 100 times as much as I have on health and nutrition. So please don't accuse me of going off on a Bible tangent!

The Bible does clearly emphasize food in relation to health. What were the first instructions God gave to man after He created him? Did He instruct man about government? About the social order? Science? Education? As important as these matters are, God passed them over and immediately instructed man about *eating!* (Genesis 1:29; 2:8-9, 16-17). Dare we say this is of no significance?

God's chosen people Israel were given vast and detailed instructions on what to eat and not to eat. Of course there are theological problems concerning how much of these instructions applied only to Israel and how much might apply to us. But on one point all can agree! These detailed instructions make it clear that *God did care what they ate!* On numerous occasions Biblical references to healing are associated with food. The very last mention of healing in the Bible makes reference to food.

> And he shewed me a pure river of water of life, clear as crystal, proceeding out of the throne of God and of the Lamb. In the midst of the street of it, and on either side of the river, was there the tree of life, which bare twelve manner of fruits, and yielded her fruit every month: and the leaves of the tree were for the healing of the nations.
>
> (Rev. 22:1-2)

Even in the Holy City, perpetual health is related to food. How can we dare continue the idea that is makes little difference about our nutritional program? God's Word seems to strongly suggest that the motto is true, "You Are What You Eat." For years I wondered why the world makes fun of natural foods and natural healing. Now I know. The world ridicules everything God does! (1 Cor. 1:18-31).

GROWING PLANTS, THE BIBLICAL SOURCE OF HEALTH

Since the brain is already programmed to repair the body, the principal secret of health is to cooperate with this divine plan of nature. If we are to help the body stay in good repair, then we must know a few things about the body. Of what is it made? This is a vital question, and the Bible gives the answer. God's Word states "And the Lord God formed man of the dust of the ground" (Gen. 2:7). Now the word "dust" here is not a term of shame. Man's shame came later when he sinned. "Dust" refers to chemical substance. So the first statement God made about the human body is that it is made of the same chemical substance as the earth. Is this not highly significant? Of the approximately 100 elements found in the earth, most of them have also been found in the human body; and some scientists suspect that almost every element on earth is present in the body, at least in minute amounts.

The healing of a damaged body requires the formation of new tissues, which of course are formed from new cells. From what are these cells made? They are made from the elements which come from the soil, of course. And how do earth elements enter the body to furnish raw material to build cells? We obviously are unable to eat dirt and thus assimilate earth nutrients! But plants can! Growing plants are God's chemical wonder workers. The growing plant absorbs earth nutrients into its own system, and then may be digesting the plant tissue receives the earth nutrients indirectly. But notice the word *indirectly*. With a few minor exceptions, there is no way man can build new life cells directly from earth's raw materials. The functioning, rebuilding, and healing of the human body is directly dependent on plant chemistry. This is God's primary law of health! Ignore it and die earlier!

Now this is not a plea for vegetarianism. I am not developing some new doctrine. I am just pointing out a simple and obvious principle of nature which we all already know but often forget to put into practice. Does the Word of God confirm the fact that human health has its basis in the plant world? Yes, there are many Biblical suggestions of this principle. In God's first instructions to newly created man, man was told to eat "the herb bearing seed" and "the fruit of a tree bearing seed" (Gen. 1:29). Notice the emphasis on seed! And previously when God described His newly created plant kingdom, in two short verses He specifically mentioned "seed" four times (Gen. 1:11-12). Don't forget this divine emphasis on seed. All plants are chemical factories that make manmade chemical factories look crude by comparison. But the seed! It's unbelievable! The chemical wonders in plant seeds stagger the imagination! Laugh it off if you like. But you'd better believe this truth which is suggested by the Word of God and confirmed by biochemistry. Later we will show how this knowledge about seeds can possibly save you from terrible suffering and an early death.

The creation story is not the only place in the Scriptures where plants and health are associated. God promised His people Israel health in the land of Canaan. When the spies went in, they reported on the crops, not the livestock (Numbers 13). King Hezekiah's almost fatal disease was cured by a preparation made from figs (2 Kings 20:7). Ezekiel the prophet foretold a day when the whole nation of Israel was to be strengthened by "a plant of reknown" (Ezek. 34:29). And the last mention of healing in the Bible—the healing of whole nations—is accomplished by the eating of fruit and leaves from a tree (Rev. 22:2).

So the Bible implies clearly that plants are the primary food and also the primary source of health. But this is no basis for strict vegetarianism. Plant food was man's original diet, but God later allowed him to add animal food (Gen. 9:2-3). Jesus approved of the eating of animal food (Luke 15:11-23), and ate fish in His resurrection body (Luke 24:36-43). But meat was eaten in Bible times primarily on festive occasions. Plant food was recognized as the primary food for man, which it is as a scientific fact. Whatever nutrients we may get from a beefsteak came from the grass and grain eaten by the cattle. So vegetation is our primary food and meat is only a secondary food, and that is not my personal prejudice. Because I am a typical American, I love to eat meat. But because I am an honest man, I must face the undeniable fact that body building materials must come to us from the earth through the channel of living plants. Both science and Scripture compel me to face this fact whether I like it or not.

So I thank God again that I have cancer, because it drove me to discover the simple fact that the primary source of health is not some man-made drug laboratory, but God's wonderful laboratory, the growing plant!

"In every thing give thanks"
(1 Thessalonians 5:18)

I can thank God for cancer, for it led me to understand this very sobering principle—

PRINCIPLE NO. 3:
MAN IS RESPONSIBLE FOR DISEASE

Sickness is such a vast human problem that it is natural for man to seek an explanation for it. Many basic causes have been theorized, and it seems that religious people are the worst at conceiving all sorts of fanciful explanations for disease, all contradictory and all supposedly from the Bible. But God's Word does not contradict itself, and most of these "religious" explanations for disease have little basis in

Scripture. Let's take a look at some of these theories. I have heard all of them promoted by good Christain people—but people who did not think clearly as they read the Scriptures.

IS GOD RESPONSIBLE FOR MAN'S DISEASE?

Some of the best people in the world make some of the worst statements in the world when disease or tragedy comes to a loved one. How often do we hear the sweet, pious, but false, attitude expressed, "It was just God's will"? What a sugar-coated insult! A precious child is crushed beneath the wheels of a car backing out of a driveway. Well meaning friends say, "God's will." That's not correct! It was man's terrible neglect! Another precious child is horribly crippled with rickets and dies much more slowly. Again well meaning neighbors say, "God's will." False again! Since the vitamin D to prevent rickets was in easy reach, this is another case of terrible human neglect. Don't blame it on God!

We must realize that God has two kinds of will. Nothing can happen without God's permission. So in that sense everything is within the *permissive* will of God. But God allows evil men, ignorant men, careless men, and even Satan to have their way sometimes—for a very short time in the light of eternity. These things are not God's *directive* will. He does not plan them and the harmful results should not be blamed on a holy and loving God. When careless men bring tragedy upon themselves, God does not cause it; He only permits it. He may even turn the tragedy around and bring good out of it (Rom. 8:28), but we still must not blame God for the tragedy!

Of course there are those occasional references in Scripture where God smites someone physically as a divine judgment. But I am not discussing that. I mean that as a general rule the Bible does not attribute human disease to a divine choice. The preponderance of evidence is to the contrary. Just look at the vast and complex healing mechanism God has placed in the human body. Look at the healing substances man has already discovered in the vegetation of the earth. The person who is fully aware of these facts will not say disease is "just the will of God." Instead he will be apalled at man's refusal to cooperate with God in His program for health. Disease is disorder or confusion, and God is not the author of confusion (1 Cor. 14:33). Don't blame God!

IS ADAM'S CURSE RESPONSIBLE FOR MAN'S DISEASE?

The Bible does teach that a curse fell on Adam because of his sin (Gen. 3:17-19). The curse was clearly said to be *death*. There is no mention of disease. But because disease and death are so closely related in our experience, many Christians have assumed that the curse includes disease. This theory leads to fatalism. If we are sick, it is Adam's fault. We can do nothing about it but humbly submit. This is only a half truth at most. Of course all the trouble in the world had its origin in Adam's sin (Rom. 5:12). But the sickness of an individual today can usually be traced directly to some present-day error of the individual or of society. Don't blame Adam for this!

To those who wish to attribute all sickness directly to Adam's sin and the curse, I would ask this question. Why did Adam live 930 years and we only live about 70? No, modern disease is not the fault of an ancient man except indirectly. Modern disease is the result of modern sin, the sin of violating God's principles of health.

It is interesting to note that Chapter 5 of the book of Genesis abounds with references to death soon after the curse of death fell on man for sin. But sickness is not mentioned until over 2000 years later (Gen. 48:1). Most of the early patriarchs apparently enjoyed good health right up to the end. They did not know disease as we know it today, yet they were sons of Adam. So our present day sickness cannot be traced back to the curse.

One more proof: Many pagan tribes live in heathen darkness and are much worse sinners *spiritually* than American Christians; nevertheless they enjoy much better health than those

American Christians. So obviously this sickness has little relation to an ancient *spiritual* problem, but is directly related to a modern *physical* problem. We are violating God's principles of health. Don't blame Adam!

IS SATAN RESPONSIBLE FOR MAN'S DISEASE?

Satan deceived Adam into sin, and so all human troubles can be traced back to the devil. But this is a long indirect path, and it is an error to blame everything *directly* on Satan. Today there is a very popular saying, "The devil made me do it!" Usually the statement is made facetiously, and the speaker seems to admit that he himself is really to blame, but he would like to blame his failures on the devil. Our attempt to blame Satan for all human illness is just this ridiculous. Satan's primary tool is deception (Gen. 3:1). He deceives man into violating God's principles of health, and then disease results. So the *direct* cause of man's disease is man. Satan is a more remote cause.

We have admitted that Satan is indirectly responsible for human sickness because he is the deceiver and no doubt he deceives many people into violating God's principles of health. Many have asked the question, "Why would the devil be interested in sickness?" This is an excellent question. The greatest thing God ever created is the human soul. So this is what Satan hates most. He directs his greatest energies at destroying man's soul. But the second greatest thing God ever created is the human body. So this is a secondary target of satanic attack. Satan likes to destroy human bodies, and bring them to death (Heb. 2:14). Why would Satan want to ruin a man's health and put him in the grave? The answer is simple. If the devil can destroy a sinner, then that sinner is lost forever to God's usefulness. This is a victory for Satan. If he can kill a Christian, he prevents that believer from winning any more souls to Christ or serving Him further in this life. The death of a human being is usually a victory for Satan. This is why the devil is deluding people to violate God's principles of health. But remember, Satan can do little to destroy us physically unless we cooperate. And if we cooperate with him, we are primarily and directly responsible for human illness. Don't blame the devil!

MAN'S TENDENCY TO DESTROY HIMSELF

Self-destruction seems to be an inherent part of human nature. I know this sounds shocking to some, but look at the evidence. The Bible plainly teaches the doctrine of human depravity (Rom. 3:10-23). Man is totally depraved. This does not mean that every person commits every imaginable sin. It means that sin has ruined every facet of human life. God said that sin would bring death (Gen. 3:19), but this referred to more than physical death, and more than eternal death in hell. Death is in every area. Death means ruin, destruction, separation from God and from God's ways. So when man became a sinner, he brought ruin into every area of human activity. Let's just mention a few.

Man has long been proud of his technology, and has pointed to it as proof of his progress. Now that same technology is drowning us in our own pollution. This is a form of death! The automobile has been one of our favorite creations. But now we realize that it is the cause of a host of major problems including air pollution, land pollution, visual pollution, noise pollution, nervous tension, under-exercise, immortality, family dissolution, crime, and many more. Now it is being called "the chariot that failed." This is a form of death!

Government, which was established by God only for the purpose of deterring crime (Gen. 9:6), has instead become a growing monster determined to control every detail of human life. This is a form of death!

Education, which should prepare man to serve his fellow man, is instead turning out a horde of rebels who can neither read nor add, but who are skilled in the art of bleeding a society which they seek to destroy. This is a form of death!

Art and music, which should lift men's souls, have in many cases become debased and vulgar, bringing out the worst in man instead of the best. This is a form of death!

These are just a few illustrations of human depravity. They help us to understand that man is depraved in every area of his life. There is no part of the social order that has not been touched by man's sin and depravity and death. It has been well said that "all of man's activities are in the realm of death." Without God, all that man touches will come to ruin and destruction. This should make it easy for us to understand that man is primarily responsible for his own disease. Man's sin and depravity are ruining his health, as shall be shown more fully as we go on.

MAN'S DESTRUCTION OF HIS OWN FOOD SUPPLY

One of the bitterest controversies in our society concerns our American diet. Is our food supply building health, or is it contributing to disease? Articles pro and con are found in almost every issue of the newspapers. Many so-called authorities in the field of nutrition argue that the American diet is the best in the world. All too often these writers are closely allied to the industrial food establishment and wish to maintain the status quo. Other nutritionists of equal competence and with no financial conflict of interest warn us of the dangers of our unnatural food supply. These latter authorities advocate a return to organic methods of food production and to a wider use of natural, unprocessed foods. So the basic question is this: which foods promote better health, natural foods or processed foods? In spite of the growing interest in natural foods in our country, I regularly run into persons who do not even know what is meant by natural foods! The answer is simple. A natural food is a food that is still in the form that God made it. A processed food is one that has been more or less changed by man. The person who is not conscious of the difference between natural foods and processed foods is not very aware of the difference between the works of God and the works of man.

As mentioned before, God makes our food to grow on plants. And we can believe He does a perfect job of it when left alone. In a secondary sense certain animals are food because they eat those plants. But here I list a few of the many processes that are widely used today to complete change our food supply from its God-given form.

Refining: For example, separating the brown part of the grain from the white part, creating an unnatural substance.

Bleaching: The use of poisonous chemicals to produce a whiter color.

Preserving: Often by use of poisonous substances to prevent growth of bacteria.

Artificial coloring and flavoring: Sometimes poisonous.

Cooking, Canning, and Pickling: Which radically changes food from its original form.

Hydrogenation: A process which changes liquid vegetable oil to solid fat, thus clogging human arteries.

Adulteration: For example, hot dogs have been found which contain only 30% meat, and 70% trash!

Hormones: Used to fatten beef cattle. Scientists and government agencies know this to be cancer-causing. But courts have protected the practice.

Commercial Fertilizer: Man-made poisonous chemicals used to fertilize crops have been found in jars of baby food.

Insecticides: Poisonous DDT sprayed on crops has been found in cow's milk.

Peeling, Shelling, Grinding: These relatively harmless processes are not totally innocent. Some foods begin to decay and even become toxic after these simple processes.

Freezing: Perhaps the least harmful of all processes.

And the list goes on and on. Man is infinitely

resourceful in finding ways to damage the food God has given him.

This raises the question: Are our processed foods equally healthful with the natural foods produced by a loving Creator? A multitude of prejudiced voices cry *yes*. But the facts to the contrary are so obvious that anyone can see them. A host of competent writers have traveled to the ends of the earth to observe the condition of primitive people who consume only natural foods. The report is always the same. Where processed foods are avoided, certain diseases are vastly lower or in some cases non-existent. And the very diseases that are almost unknown among these peoples are the same ones that head the list of killers and cripplers in our society: cancer, high blood pressure, stroke, diabetes, and arthritis. These are the *chronic* diseases, they do not usually go away by themselves, and they cannot be transmitted to another person. All these diseases are related to the body metabolism. No metabolic disease in history has ever been conquered except through *nutrition*. On the other hand, the infectious diseases, which are due to invading organisms, sometimes strike these primitive peoples as badly or worse than in our land. To put it another way, medical science in our country has made considerable progress in combatting infectious diseases, but has made almost no progress against the chronic metabolic diseases. This is due to our degenerating American food supply and to the refusal of orthodox medicine to face the seriousness of this problem.

Is this fact surprising? Not at all! The believer who understands the Word of God is not surprised that God's natural foods are superior to man's processed foods. God's ways are as superior to man's ways as the heavens are higher than the earth (Isa. 55:9). Also we should not be surprised that man often destroys his own food supply. This is consistent with man's depravity. Man's depraved nature leads him to pursue error in every facet of his life.

URBAN LIFE, THE ENEMY OF HEALTH

One may rightly ask, "Isn't food processing essential to some degree?" There is no excuse for the enormous excess in modern food processing, especially the refining which removes essential nutrients and the use of poisons as preservatives. Even in our modern complex society, we could find ways to consume more natural foods and to avoid extreme processing. But the basic problem that brought on the processing binge is the urbanization of our society. And this again is at its root a spiritual problem. Most Bible students are aware that God originally planned for man to live close to the soil. He was to be basically a farmer (Gen. 1:28; 9:1). The Lord apparently never gave man permission to crowd up in cities, and almost every movement toward urban life was associated with evil (Gen. 4:16-17; 11:1-9).

Notice the many ways that city life is destructive to human health. Urban dwellers generally do not have access to fresh natural foods. Some processing seems to be necessary in order to preserve the foods for shipment to the cities. But once the processing begins, there seems to be no end to it. Cities create sewage disposal problems and problems of air pollution, industrial waste, and water contamination. These are of course disease-producing. Contagious diseases spread more rapidly where people are crowded in close contact. City dwellers generally get less exercise than those who till the soil. Urban living tends toward a fast pace of life where there is little time for the things of the spirit. City life with its crowding creates tension, nervousness, personal conflict, class conflict, frustration, violence, and crime.

This list could go on almost indefinitely. But this is enough to remind us that man is primarily responsible for most of his own problems, including disease. For centuries, great preachers of the Word have warned us of the spiritual danger of city life, but the world laughed at them. But today most sociologists recognize that urbanization lies at the root of all social ills, including strife, crime, pollution, and disease.

To those who reply that the great Apostle Paul spent most of his time in the great population centers, please be reminded that he went there as a missionary to those who were away from God. He did not go there to enjoy the thrills of urban life.

I must say again that I am glad that I have cancer. It motivated me to think and study about the mystery of sickness. Now I understand the basic cause of my disease. I am partly responsible for it because for over half a century I ignorantly violated some of God's laws of health. But the society in which I live is also partly responsible for my cancer, because that society placed before me an artificial food supply and encouraged me to violate God's health principles. I'm glad I learned the truth; now I won't blame my disease on God. I will not blame it on father Adam or the curse. I will not even blame it on the devil except indirectly. I am sorry that man is to blame for most of his sickness. But since it is true, I am glad I learned it!

"In every thing give thanks"
(1 Thessalonians 5:18)

I can thank God for cancer, because it led me to understand this basic physiological principle—

PRINCIPLE NO. 4: NO ONE CAN HEAL YOU BUT YOURSELF

I feel that this chapter will be misunderstood by some individuals in the healing professions. But the things written here are not intended to knock the medical doctor or those in related fields. The purpose is to help the reader see the health professions in the proper perspective, in relation to God and to the total healing program. The Word of God on more than one occasion warns of the danger of placing too much confidence in the physician to the neglect of other aspects of health and healing (2 Chron. 16:12; Mark 5:26). To prove my absolute fairness in this matter I will sound the same warning concerning the religious profession (of which I am a part) as I do concerning the medical profession. No person can afford to leave his spiritual health entirely in the hands of a minister. The minister may be able to help, but the individual is responsible for putting his own soul in proper relation to God. A professional man of religion can be mistaken, he can be ignorant, he can even be greedy and dishonest like any other man. The same is true of the professional man of medicine. So the individual must assume the primary responsibility for putting his own body in proper relation to God. This writer has been amazed at the number of Christians who would never accept the idea of an infallible religious profession, yet who have always assumed the infallibility of the medical profession. Why should we think that medical men are free from the same weaknesses that plague other members of Adam's fallen race?

So I am not knocking the physician, just facing the fact that the medical organization is not God. Therefore the individual is most foolish who assumes that his health is being well cared for by some group of scientists in some distant place. The primary responsibility for your physical well-being rests squarely on your own shoulders!

THE BODY DOES THE HEALING

If you are ever healed, you will heal yourself. This is true in a very real and practical sense. As mentioned in a preceding section, your body was designed by the Creator to heal and repair itself. Like an intricate computer, the brain directs every organ and every cell in the work of combatting disease and rebuilding healthy tissues. Obviously then, each individual heals himself. No ordinary human being can heal another person. Jesus Christ, the God-man, is the only exception. Since He is the Creator and the Sustainer of the creation (Col. 1:16), He can touch and heal others. In fact, all healing is from Him. This is a divine principle. But on the human side, your own body does the healing.

This points out clearly that professional practitioners *do not heal!* God heals, your body heals, but doctors do not heal. All a physician can do is to cooperate with God. If the doctor cooperates with God's principles of healing, then he can facilitate healing. But if the doctor violates any of these principles, he can do harm and prevent healing. He can set the broken bone straight or crooked. He can prescribe the right medicine or the wrong. He can recommend the right kind of nutrition or the wrong kind. He can hinder. The best he can do is cooperate, but he cannot heal. God does all the healing, but he uses your own body as the instrument to accomplish this healing.

This reminds us of a bit of medical philosophy that is only a half-truth. It is often said in medical circles that "He who is his own doctor has a food for a patient." This is partly true. But remember that a half-truth is also half-lie. And nothing could be more dangerous than a half-lie. If we are thinking of self-medication using dangerous drugs, then probably one should not be his own physician. But if we are thinking of cooperating with God in the maintaining of health, then each individual *must be his own physician*. This is a Christian obligation. Since the body of the believer is the temple of the Holy Spirit (1 Cor. 6:19), then the Christian must assume the responsibility of caring for this temple. He cannot shrug off this duty and assume that a medical establishment has everything under control. Only you can heal yourself! No other mortal being can do it for you! What will happen if you refuse to accept this responsibility?

I have many friends in the healing profession for whom I have the greatest admiration. But it is also true that for twenty-five years a series of physicians were never able to give me any information on some chronic health problems. But when I decided to assume this responsibility myself, a little reading in some health literature produced many answers which I could never get from professional sources. In my case, I would be either dead or an invalid today if I had not, to a certain extent, become my own physician.

Even though I still use the services of physicians, the primary responsibility for my health is mine. Only I can heal myself. If I get sick and go to a doctor, then to some degree I have failed in my responsibility.

GOD'S PRINCIPLES OF HEALTH ARE IMPERSONAL

There is a danger that the child of God may develop a false confidence concerning his physical condition. He may assume that the laws of health do not apply to him. He can live as he pleases; God will take care of him and give him health. Perhaps the warning of 1 Cor. 10:12 is appropriate here, "Let him that thinketh he standeth take heed lest he fall."

God in His infinite grace may sometimes overrule the foolishness of man. He may sometimes give a measure of health in spite of self-abuse. This is just an illustration of the fact that God's grace is greater than human sin. But no one can presume on such grace of God! Outside of an occasional miracle of grace, God's laws of health are inexorable. The wages of sin is death! This is true in the spiritual realm and in the physical. To violate God's laws of health is to invite death.

These principles are impersonal. God is no respector of persons. It matters not if one is Christian or pagan, good nutrition promotes health and poor nutrition promotes disease.

Whether one is spiritual or worldly, proper exercise encourages health and no exercise encourages the breakdown of health. Whether a person knows it or doesn't know it, emotional tension still promotes disease just as emotional harmony encourages health. These laws work. They work for all. They work whether we know it or not.

The practical lesson is this: We cannot leave our bodily health up to chance. We cannot presume on the goodness of God to keep us well while we violate His principles. His laws of health are working in our bodies. Ignorance is no excuse. We are responsible to cooperate with our own body healing. What will we do about it?

MANY TYPES OF "HEALERS" ARE SUCCESSFUL

There are many types of so-called healers in our world. Each individual usually has certain types of healers in which he has confidence, and other types which he is quite sure are quacks and charlatans. But the next person, just as intelligent and just as godly, has an entirely different line-up of "true" and "false" healers. But the shocking truth is that every type of healer is having successes and every type is having failures. Many of us would be amazed to find how close the success ratio is among different healers.

Let us list here some of the various types of

healers who are currently engaged in the healing arts of the world today:

Medical Doctor

Osteopath

Chiropractor

Psychiatrist

Psychologist

Naturopath (uses such natural means as nutrition, exercise, etc.)

Healing evangelist, or faith healer

Christian Science practitioner

Thought control cultist

Spiritualist (or spirit medium)

Witch doctor.

No doubt you can point to some of these in which you have great confidence. Probably there are others on the list that you would condemn. The orthodox Christian will object to some on theological grounds. But be that as it may, that does not alter the fact that *all of these types of healers are having successes!*

Some of my readers are no doubt shocked. Here I am, a Bible-believing Baptist preacher, a fundamentalist, admitting that a heathen witch doctor sometimes has healing successes. I may not like it, but that doesn't change the fact that it happens! How could a heathen witch doctor, without the knowledge of the true God and probably worshipping the devil, influence anyone to be healed? Simple! If he knowingly or ignorantly cooperates with any of God's laws of healing, he will get results. Remember, God's laws are impersonal. Many witch doctors use herbs, and in some cases the herb contains the substance needed for healing. But more important than that, if the witch doctor or any other practitioner convinces the patient that he is going to get better, he probably will. There is no area in which psychology works more powerfully than in the matter of healing. When the patient has a good mental attitude, all his glands function more efficiently, his secretions of vital hormones and enzymes are improved, and this promotes physical health. All so-called healers agree on one point—that a hopeful mental attitude promotes healing. And it makes no difference whether that good mental attitude was induced by a scholarly M.D. or by an ignorant witch doctor; it helps in either case. This argument does not imply that all healers are *equally* successful, merely that they all do have some degree of success. This points out again the fact that the body does the healing. None of these "healers" heal. But all of them can to some degree influence the patient mentally or physically, and can thereby encourage the body to heal itself.

YOU CAN'T DEPEND ENTIRELY ON THE DOCTOR

I am well aware of the great advances that have been made in the medical professions. I am thankful for the successes that have been achieved in combatting infectious diseases and parasites, the heroic rebuilding of bodies following major injuries, and other great accomplishments of medical science. I am also painfully aware of the dismal failure of organized medicine to come up with any prevention or highly successful treatment of the *chronic* disease—such as cancer, diabetes, high blood pressure, stroke, heart attack, and arthritis. There are the great killers and cripplers in our country; and in spite of our vast medical machine, instead of being solved these medical problems are on the increase. One does not have to be overly critical to conclude that American medicine is a failure in this area. The facts are there. In general, we can have a considerable degree of confidence in the medical profession in the treatment of infections and injuries. But we can have little confidence in their ability to promote health, to prevent disease, or to treat chronic diseases. Here we give the four reasons why we cannot leave these areas up to the professionals.

First, all chronic diseases result from improper body metabolism—in other words, defective body chemistry or just plain poor nutrition. The average person imagines that a physician is an expert in nutrition. Nothing could be farther from the truth. Medical science and nutrition are two separate fields. American medical schools teach almost nothing in this area. Only a few class periods are usually given to this extremely vital field. Our medical schools are oriented toward pathology and disease rather than toward health. The medical student is given a cadaver to dissect, and from this he may learn to discover certain pathological conditions. But how much does he study healthy bodies? The academic emphasis is not on health, how to preserve health, or how to cooperate with nature in the maintenance of health. The emphasis is on discovering what organ is diseased and how to cut it out. The basic philosophy is negative rather than positive. Of course this is a part of our culture. We do not pay doctors to keep us from getting sick. We go ahead and make ourselves sick and then pay the doctor to cut out the damaged part.

In many parts of the world and in many periods of history, physicians have been employed to study health, and to supervise the patient in preventing disease. This is a far better philosophy. But in general, American doctors are not highly interested in preventing chronic diseases. In one American city of about a million population, I was able to find only one medical doctor who would openly announce that he specialized in the field of preventive medicine. This is due to several factors. Perhaps not enough people are willing to pay for prevention. The schools do not emphasize prevention. And of course, promoting health does not furnish the pride and prestige that is afforded to the doctors that treat the disease. There seems to be something glamorous about treating terrible diseases, even if the disease could have been prevented and even if the treatment fails. In fact, the more impossible the cure, the more glamorous. Maybe our whole society has become pathological in its thinking. We seem to get more satisfaction out of disease than we do from health.

The second reason why we cannot trust our health entirely to medical men is this: they are sick too. If medical doctors knew how to keep people healthy, then surely they and their families would enjoy an abundance of health and vitality. Let's see if that is the case. Recently a carefully controlled study was made to determine the health of American physicians and their families. Over five hundred doctors in all parts of America were studied, along with their families. It was a typical cross section of the medical profession. Most of the doctors were in their thirties or forties, certainly not old. Here are the results: 10% had already had cancer, 12% had anemia, 21% had hay fever, 24% had major surgery, 30% were overweight, and 41% had hemorrhoids! The conclusion is inescapable: the medical profession in our country does not know how to stay healthy! How then can they keep us healthy? The proverb that was so frequently used in Bible times is still a wise bit of advice, "Physician, heal thyself." Until our medical men can learn something about health, we are most unwise to leave our health entirely in their hands.

There is a third reason why we cannot leave our health entirely up to organized medicine. Medical men are just human, not gods. They too are members of Adam's fallen race, just like the rest of us. They have the same weaknesses as lawyers, or clergymen, or anyone else. They can become puffed up with pride. They can become greedy and selfish. They can look out for their own vested interests, just like other people. And medical organizations intensify this problem. The Bible teaches that the world works against God. The truth is unpleasant but inescapable. When men of the world form organizations, they do not promote the work of God. Whether it be a labor union, a political party, a corporation, a religious denomination, or a medical association, the result is the same. The members are pressured more and more to conform. They are no longer free men, but part of a powerful machine. Medical organizations do not exist to promote the welfare of the patients. They exist to look out for the economic welfare of the physicians. And as a result even Christian doctors often report that they are pressured to follow principles that violate their own consciences. They must use the same methods that other doctors use or suffer serious persecution. The physician I mentioned earlier who was the only one in his city practicing preventive medicine was for years threatened by his local medical society. They disapproved of any doctor using nutrition extensively in the treatment of patients. Because of this organized worldly pressure that hinders the physician from seeking to cooperate with nature and God, we cannot leave our health entirely in their hands.

There is yet a fourth reason why no informed and intelligent person will trust his life and health entirely to the healing profession. And this is the saddest reason of all. For several hundred years, organized medicine has resisted nearly every discovery that promised to revolutionize medical science and to save multitudes of lives. In many cases the discoverer was ridiculed, harassed, and persecuted almost to death. In general, the new discovery was opposed if it was a simple remedy or if it threatened the pride or economic welfare of the medical establishment. Details of this opposition will be given in the next chapter. We are most foolish if we believe that this problem no longer exists. This type of opposition is still with us in increasing power.

Your personal physician may be a dedicated and honest man, but he is part of a machine. He is not a completely free man. He usually believes the propaganda that is fed to him. He must practice what other doctors practice or he may lose his license. For these reasons, it is obvious that I cannot abandon my responsibility to care for the temple of the Holy Spirit. I may use a medical doctor, but I must not let the medical establishment use me. I am responsible to learn how to care for my own health. I must cooperate with God in this matter.

DON'T DEPEND ENTIRELY ON YOUR FAITH IN MIRACLES

Some of my friends in the medical profession may resent the preceding section a bit because of misunderstanding. If you are one of these, then you can relax a while, because in this section some of my religious friends are going to resent me a bit, also because of misunderstanding. Just as a distorted emphasis can be given to the healing professions, so likewise a distorted emphasis can be given to the place of miracles in healing. Now I'm sure that this statement will be misinterpreted! Can you imagine an old-fashioned Baptist preacher of conservative and fundamental convictions making such a statement? Now get me straight! I know of a certainty that Jehovah is a God of miracles. He is the Ruler of nature. He is the Author of all natural laws and He can and does set aside natural law when He sees fit. He is the God of the natural and also of the supernatural. I believe in miracles. I know miracles take place, and Christians should expect them.

But on the other hand, I also know that under certain conditions an emphasis on miracles can be evil. "An evil and adulterous generation seeketh after a sign" (Matt. 12:39). Is it not evil to ask God to solve our problem by a supernatural method when He has already given a natural solution to the problem? For example, suppose a farmer has a great stream of water flowing through his fields, and a little bit of work could divert the current in such a way as to irrigate all of his crops. But he refuses to do this. Instead he prays that God will burst open the bowels of the earth and let water rise up from the depths to flood his fields. You say ridiculous! Yes, but I have known many persons, Christians, but confused Christians, who do just that. They refuse to follow a few simple rules of natural health which God has given us. Then when they get sick, while still ignoring God's natural means of healing, they cry long and loud for a miracle of healing. I have seen men develop lung cancer from smoking, then keep on smoking while they assure me that God is going to heal them by a miracle. This preacher has seen scores of Christians die after professing loudly for days that God was going to heal them by a miracle. Now this does not imply at all that God cannot or does not perform supernatural acts of healing. What it does illustrate is this: we have no right to scorn God's natural way of healing and then demand a supernatural way of healing. We cannot presume on the goodness of God while disobeying the principles He has ordained.

This raises a question: Why did the Lord Jesus

declare that it was sometimes evil to seek after a miracle? I suggest an explanation. To receive a miracle sometimes is quite exciting, it contains the element of entertainment, it tickles our fancy, it projects us into the limelight, it boosts our ego, it can make us boastful and proud! Are we not somebody special? Have we not been chosen to share in a supernatural experience? Big deal! On the other hand, to quietly learn God's simple laws of health and healing and to cooperate with these laws—this is not glamorous at all. Far from it! We are more likely to be rejected as a health nut!

In the case of my own healing, many of my Christian friends felt I had experienced a *supernatural* healing. But the evidence I had seen indicated to me that it was more likely a *natural* healing. To me that makes it no less wonderful. Less exciting perhaps, but no less wonderful. I believe that the same healing is available to anyone else who would follow the same procedures. In one way this is more wonderful than a supernatural event. What God showed me could be passed on to others, but a miraculous healing could not. My healing was from God and it was in answer to prayer. God gave me wisdom and understanding to follow His laws. But when I announced to my friends that my healing was natural rather than miraculous, some of them resented it. They wanted the kick of being associated with a miracle. They were not interested in natural foods, vitamins, mineral, enzymes, proteins, or any other "health nut" ideas. They wanted a miracle!

Thank God He answered my prayer and gave me sense enough to cooperate with Him. It is great to believe in a God that can overrule the laws of nature and perform the unusual. But I believe it is just as wonderful, perhaps more so, to know a God who regularly, seven days a week, all over the world, promotes health and healing by clearly established and uniform principles. So don't wait for a miracle. Learn to cooperate with God now!

DON'T DEPEND ENTIRELY ON PRAYER

This section is closely related to the preceding section, but we can add a few additional ideas. Prayer is vital. Christians *must* pray. But there are times when prayer alone may be displeasing to God. Someone has said we need to put feet to our prayers. That means as we pray we also obey what God shows us to do. We are willing to be active and to let God work through us. Imagine a missionary who prays for the heathen around him but who declines to give them the gospel. Will God honor his prayers? How about a farmer who prays for a good harvest but will not plow or cultivate or do anything else to promote a good harvest? Will God honor his prayers? How about a sick person who prays for health, but he refuses to eat natural foods, continues to stuff himself with refined and preserved man-made poisons, and will not exercise or follow any of God's principles of good health? Will God honor his prayers? You see, God *can* function without our cooperation, but He usually does not do so. As a general rule, He expects our cooperation along with our prayers.

Did you know there are times when it is wrong to pray? Joshua was ordered by the Lord to get up off his face and stop praying (Josh. 7:10). Why? Joshua had not yet done what he knew he should do. This is a great spiritual principle. It may be wrong for me to ask God for health when I have not yet done what I know I should do about my health. God's word tells us that obedience is better than sacrifice (1 Sam. 15:22). Since sacrifice and prayer are closely related religious activities, we might conclude that in some cases obedience is better than prayer. This is not to minimize the power of prayer, but to emphasize that we cannot expect God to do everything while we stubbornly refuse to do our part. We need to pray, but we also need to understand *how* God answers prayer. He may not intervene in our sickness by a direct act. He may not touch the body and cause a special healing. Instead He may give us some new insights and some new understandings so that we can cooperate with His natural healing methods. That's what He did in my case. So sick friend, have you been begging God to heal you by some *special* method? Perhaps He has other plans for you. Perhaps He wants you to be healed by His *regular* methods, the ones He has used for thousands of years to heal millions of people. Wouldn't that be good enough?

OTHER FACTORS IN HEALTH AND DISEASE

Our discussion so far might create the impression that nutrition is the only factor in health and disease. Of course this is not the case. But nutrition is vitally important to our discussion because it is the biggest factor under the control of the individual. Both world-wide experience and the suggestions of Scripture place food at the top of the list in any program of personal health. But there are many other factors, some under the control of the individual and some not. For example, the layman has very little control over diseases caused by genetic or congenital defects. He may be able to do little about infectious epidemics. But even in these cases, the properly nourished individual has far greater powers of resistance and recuperation.

There are some factors other than nutrition over which we do have much control, and which make a great contribution to personal health.

Exercise. The Word of God tells us that "the life of the flesh is in the blood" (Lev. 17:11). Moses proclaimed this fact about 1500 B.C., but only in recent years has medical science realized the importance of this principle. It is not enough for proper food to be placed in the stomach. This food must be assimilated and carried by the blood stream to every cell in the body. The better the flow of blood, the better is the nutritional environment of the cells. We need to see exercise not primarily as a means to develop muscles. Far more important is the matter of increased respiration and circulation that results from regular rhythmical exercise. No doubt a large portion of our degenerative diseases result from an inadequate blood supply which in turn is due to our sedentary way of life.

Emotions. It has been estimated by many authorities that fully one-half of the hospital beds in our country are occupied by patients whose illness is not the result of any physical pathology. Instead the illness is emotional in its origin, although the physical body does become involved. These are the psychosomatic illnesses, and they continue to be on the increase in our country. How do improper emotions harm the body? One way is in the disturbance of the glands and other organs. Fear, hate, or anxiety can stop or slow down the functions of the glands. Thus the body is deprived of much-needed hormones and enzymes. Physical harm results. Some of the more common physical conditions resulting from emotional stress are indigestion, diarrhea, high blood pressure, rashes, and allergies. When prolonged these can develop into colitis, stroke, or heart attack. As will be shown later, there is growing evidence that certain enzymes play a part in the prevention of cancer. But emotional stress can slow down the glands that produce these enzymes. So our cancer epidemic in this country is partly due to our tension-producing culture, although its primary cause is undoubtedly our unnatural food habits. Does the Bible mention emotions in relation ot health? Yes, many times. The writer of the Proverbs stated that "there is he that speaketh like the piercings of a sword, but the tongue of the wise is health" (Prov. 12:18). Expressed in modern terminology, this simply states that our conversation can promote health or tear down health. I wonder how many children are enjoying abundant health and vitality because the parents create a pleasant and healthy emotional climate that encourages proper functioning of the child's endocrine system! And how many children are chronically ill because the glands and certain other organs are paralyzed by the constant anger and hatred in the home? I have seen dedicated but ignorant Christians scream at their children at meal time, slap them, and force them to eat foods which were distasteful to them. Shame! No wonder the "bad" child vomited up his food or had an attack of diarrhea or hives. Far better to eat no food than to eat in an environment of tension. "Better is a dinner of herbs where love is, than a stalled ox and hatred therewith" (Prov. 15:17).

Want to stay healthy? Then avoid emotional tension. Maintain a happy mental attitude.

No doubt many will say "How?" "How can I stop my habit of fear and worry and anger?" It is simply a matter of trust in a loving Heavenly Father.

> Be careful for nothing, but in everything, by prayer and supplication with thanksgiving, let your requests be made known unto God. And the peace of God, which passeth all understanding, shall keep your hearts and minds through Christ Jesus. (Phil. 4:6-7)

The Christian has a moral responsibility to maintain an attitude of peace, and thus to promote his physical well-being.

Pollution. Another factor in health and disease which is to some degree under our control is the matter of pollution. We suffer from air pollution, water pollution, soil pollution, food pollution, noise pollution, and many others. Some of this is beyond the control of the individual, but much of it we could avoid with a little common sense and effort. We can avoid exhaust fumes as much as possible, and we can eat more fresh foods and thus avoid the deadly poisons used to "preserve" our processed foods. We can cry out against the crime of putting deadly flouride in our city's water supply. We can stay away from contact with chemicals as much as possible. I have seen a list of some two hundred man-made chemicals that are suspected of being carcinogenic (cancer-causing) by an agency of the U.S. Government. It would be wise then to view all unnatural chemical substances with suspicion and to avoid contact with them as much as possible.

Does the Word of God make any reference to the problem of pollution? Yes, many times—at least indirectly. The entire tone of Scripture from Genesis to Revelation suggests that man's sin and depravity cause him to damage the things God has made. In the last few years scientists have expressed surprise and horror at the way "civilized" man has polluted his own environment. But this fact has not surprised the Bible student at all. We knew it was coming. The Apostle Peter in one of his letters tells of a future day when God will purify the earth with a great fire (2 Pet. 3:3-12). This divine cleansing will destroy all of the consequences of man's sin, including pollution. If God wants a clean world, so should we.

Therefore, we do have a responsibility to take care of the temple of the Holy Spirit. We cannot delegate this responsibility to anyone else, however capable. We must realize that no professional can heal the body. The body is the only thing that can heal the body. This is a solemn fact, and places squarely on our shoulders the responsibility to know and follow God's laws of health. Someone will say "How can I learn how to care for my health? It's all so complicated." Not really, the basic principles are quite simple. Literature on nature's way of health is abundant. Hundreds of writers and scores of publishers are turning out an ever increasing supply of books and pamphlets on natural health. You might want to join the increasing millions of Americans who have made their health food store their health library. Get a basic book on natural foods and begin there. You can go as far as you like in this field of research. Each publication will refer you to other publications, and your knowledge will begin to grow. Similar information might be available in some libraries. But a word of caution. Just because a book professes to deal with health is no proof that it *really* deals with health. If it does not promote natural foods, then it is not cooperating with God's way and is of little value to you!

One of my life's greatest discoveries is this simple fact: no one can heal me but myself. I am glad I learned this, even if it did take cancer to drive me to this discovery.

"In every thing give thanks"
(1 Thessalonians 5:18)

I can thank God for cancer, for it led me to become aware of this sad historical principle—

PRINCIPLE NO. 5: THE WORLD OPPOSES GOD'S WAY OF HEALING

This chapter may be shocking to some of my readers, but it will be no surprise to those who are thoroughly grounded in the basic teachings of the Word of God. Before we can proceed, we must make sure that the reader clearly understands the meaning of the word *world*. The

English word *world* as found in the New Testament may have a variety of meanings. The most common Greek term is *cosmos*, and the usual meaning of this word is order, arrangement, or organization. The *cosmos* then usually refers to mankind organized in his social institutions.

THE BIBLE DESCRIPTION OF THE WORLD

We are taught to praise man's social order and to have great admiration for our social institutions. The Word of God, however, presents an entirely different view of the world. Almost invariably the context indicates a negative moral attitude toward the world. In no case is the world praised. Plainly then the term implies mankind organized into societies and institutions, but with God left out.

The principles upon which this world is founded are clearly spelled out in 1 John 2:15-17. They are "the lust of the flesh, the lust of the eyes, and the pride of life." In other words, sensuality, greed, and pride. These principles are plainly said to be not of God.

Who is the leader of this present world-system? The Lord Jesus Christ plainly identified Satan as the prince of this world (John 12:31). The Bible says that every person is by nature under the control of Satan unless he has been saved by Jesus Christ (John 8:44; Eph. 2:1-3; 1

John 3:10). Satan can control men much better when he can organize them into groups. He began this system of world organization at the tower of Babel (Gen. 11:1-9), and will complete his program of world control in the coming Great Tribulation (Rev. 13:1-18). These Bible facts need not imply that every human group on earth is totally wicked and that no man-made institution ever did anything beneficial. What is clearly taught is that every man-made institution is *potentially* evil, for Satan can get control of it no matter how noble its goals may appear at first. Experience has shown that human institutions tend to become more evil with the passing of time, and the larger and more powerful they become the more dangerous they are.

What is the attitude of this present world toward God and Christ? Jesus said that the world hates Him and His followers (John 7:7; 14:17; 15:18; 17:14). The reason for this hatred is non-conformity. The true Christian is not of this world (John 17:16), and a true church is the one institution on the earth that is not based on the philosophy of this world. But even true Christians are subject to the social pressures of the world and may be influenced by it. Of course the world often feigns admiration for Christ while viciously opposing His principles.

What should be the attitude of the Christian toward the world? He must be separate from it (2 Cor. 6:17)—that is, refuse to accept its philosophies, principles, and goals. The world will try to make him conform , but he must resist this pressure (Rom. 12:1-2) and permit Christ to completely transform his mind, or way of thinking. If the Christian follows the teaching of any social institution, no matter how prestigious or noble in its appearance, then he has substituted the leadership of man for the leadership of God. And he will not find the leadership of God (John 5:44). This holds true whether we are talking of a religious denominational headquarters, a medical society, or any other man-made institution. What does God think of our world, our much vaunted social order? God views all its wisdom (philosophy) as foolishness! (1 Cor. 1:18-31). So much for the general principles of our present world-system. Now let us examine certain facets of our social order in the light of these principles.

THE WORLD OF RELIGION

Let us look first at the world of religion. We must realize that religion is not salvation, and religion does not necessarily please God. Almost every time the word *religion* appears in the New Testament it is in a bad moral sense. It is one thing to be religious and quite another thing to be a Christian, a born-again child of God through faith in Jesus Christ. So we are talking about the religious world, not necessarily true Christians.

The Scriptures clearly reveal several basic principles that are generally true in the world of religion:

Satan is the head of the religious world, except of course that small segment that is truly born into God's family through faith in Jesus Christ (John 8:44; 1 Cor. 10:20).

The majority of persons in the world of religion are on the wrong road, the broad road that leads to destruction (Matt. 7:13-14). Of course the majority can gain vast political power even though they are false—for example, the National Council of Churches.

The evil leadership in the world of religion rejects God's way of salvation through Jesus Christ, and substitutes man's way, salvation through religion or morality (Jer. 2:13; Acts 7:51).

The corrupt leadership in the world of religion, seeking to promote their own vested interests, seeks to destroy the competition, and persecute those who stand up for the truth (Acts 7:52).

These evil persecutors, through self-delusion, can even imagine that they are serving God when they persecute the truth (John 16:2).

The lesser officials in the religious hierarchy cannot follow the truth of God as long as they seek to please the men at the top (John 12:42-43).

It was this loyalty to a human institution that caused the crucifixion of Jesus. The common people had seen abundant evidence that Jesus

Christ was what He claimed to be, the Son of God. But the religious rulers wanted to destroy Him because He was a threat to their economic and political power (Matt. 27:18). And the powerful influence of the leaders coerced the common people to reject Him in spite of the evidence they had seen (John 7:46-48).

The reader will do well to ponder these principles thoroughly. They sound an ominous warning about the danger of loyalty to any man-made institution. Loyalty to this present evil world, or loyalty to any segment of it, can place you in the position of fighting against Almighty God Himself. Better be careful!

A COMPARISON OF THE RELIGIOUS WORLD AND THE MEDICAL WORLD

I can almost hear some of my readers exclaim at this point that the Bible only rebukes the *religious* world for opposing God, and that it does not condemn other facets of society. But Scripture plainly teaches that "the world by wisdom knew not God" (1 Cor. 1:21). The whole cosmos was and is against Him. He was opposed by the religious world, the political world, the military world, the entertainment world, the philosophical world, the whole world. In fact, the Jewish writers of Scripture did not analyze the world into segments as we do. It was seen as a world—and a world whose purposes worked against the purposes of God.

Let us see if the medical world could be expected to cooperate with God better than the religious world. We agree that God's greatest creation is the human soul, and therefore Satan's primary opposition is in this area. But is it not true that God's second greatest creation is the human body? And would not Satan also be interested in opposing God's work in this area? Doesn't Satan hate the human body, just as truly as he hates the human soul? Would he not seek to gain power in a medical organization the same as he would in a religious organization? Would he not seek to work through the American Medical Association the same as he would try to work through the National Council of Churches? These statements will come as somewhat of a shock to some of my fundamental, Bible-believing Christian friends. They realize that the National Council of Churches is looked upon by the government as the "official" voice of religion in this country. They also realize that this organization is led primarily by men who reject the claims of Jesus Christ as the eternal Son of God. These friends of mine know that the religious hierarchy in America is heavily weighted against God, and that the faithful preacher is in the minority and is often ridiculed as a "nut." Yet these same friends of mine have absolute confidence in our medical hierarchy. They imagine that the official decrees of this medical hierarchy are absolute truth. And they also imagine that any physician who departs from the rules of the hierarchy must be a quack. Now look at the absurdity of this. Christian people know the religious world is devilish, but they imagine the medical world to be saintly! Strange that Christians are cautious about believing preachers, but totally gullible about believing doctors! If you are one of these I would like to ask you a question. What makes you think that the organized world of doctors is more trustworthy than the organized world of preachers? Do you really expect the medical world to be better than the religious world? Let's not be stupid any longer! Let's use the brains God gave us and realize that God meant what He said when He warned us that there is evil in the whole world, all of it! The medical world is not exempt from this Bible principle!

THE SHAMEFUL HISTORY OF THE MEDICAL PROFESSION

Today there are several million Americans who know full well that certain elements in our medical-drug complex are opposing simple and natural means of preventing disease. Yet there are other millions who have never heard of this and who cannot believe it when they first hear it. How many times I have been present in a conversation where it was mentioned that a certain vitamin or other natural substance was helpful in preventing a certain disease. Then I have heard the very "brilliant" remark that surely this could not be true because if it were true then all the doctors would be using it. The speaker always imagines that he has brought forth the ultimate in human logic and has forever dispensed of the idea. Such abysmal ignorance is almost nauseating! How can intelligent human beings be unaware that certain elements in organized medicine have consistently opposed natural healing and medical progress for centuries? Let us look at a few examples.

In 1535, the famous French explorer Jacques Cartier was exploring the St. Lawrence River, and his crew was dying of scurvy. An Indian showed him how to treat the surviving men with a drink made from tree bark. The results were immediate and thorough! Today we know that the active ingredient of the tree bark was vitamin C. But the European medical establishment opposed this treatment until 1795. In the 260 years of "scientific" opposition over two million sailors died a terrible death of scurvy—*after the cure was known!* Why? This new treatment struck at the pride, the prejudice, and the pocketbooks of the medical establishment! This was exactly the same set of principles that caused the crucifixion of Jesus!

In 1543, the Flemish anatomist Andreas Vesalius published his monumental work, *De Humanis Corporis Fabrica*. For this great contribution to medical science he is today called the founder of modern anatomy. But in his own day he met powerful opposition from all the great medical authorities of Europe. Why? Because his new teachings upset all their established ideas. His discoveries required the abandonment of previous theories and practices. Because of vested interests, the medical schools of Europe opposed and ridiculed him. However, now we know that he was right and they were wrong. We may well wonder how many surgical patients were needlessly butchered because the medical world refused to accept the truth?

In 1628, the British physician William Harvey published his treatise which explained the workings of the circulatory system. Previously it had been believed that the liver constantly manufactured a fresh supply of blood. Draining off the stale and used-up blood was a common medical practice. But Harvey showed that the blood recirculates and is used again. Today his work on this subject is classed as the greatest medical treatise of all time. But in his day? He was abused and rejected by the medical authorities. History had recorded the fact that these medical politicians ignored the plain evidence and stubbornly chose to remain blind.

In 1799, George Washington lay ill with a sore throat. Of course, the finest medical men available were called in. He was heavily bled four times in an effort to heal him. This was consensus medicine (standard practice) at that time. Ofcourse the treatment failed. The death certificate officially stated that he died of a respiratory infection. But that is a lie! A thing can be "official" and still be false! George Washington was slaughtered by an organized medical establishment that refused to look at the truth! Dr. Harvey had shown scientific proof 171 years earlier that bleeding the patient was a harmful practice. And Moses had revealed 33 centuries earlier that "the life of the flesh is in the blood" (Lev. 17:11). There was no excuse for this needless killing of the father of our country! But time-honored medical practices must be followed! Facts are not important! According to modern legal-medical practice, the family of George Washington could not successfully sue the physician because he was following consensus medicine. But if he had *not* bled the president, he would be subject to a malpractice suit because he was not following consensus medicine and would therefore be a "quack." You see, standard practice must prevail— scientific facts and the Word of God notwithstanding! The last words of the dying president to his physician were, "I thank you for your attentions." He thanked the man who ignored the Bible, ignored science, followed standard medical practice, and took his life! I wonder how often today a patient is lost because the physician refuses to cooperate with God's principles of natural healing? I have good reason to believe I have seen several such cases. Yet the patient and the family praise and thank the killer! Did I hear someone say, "That's too strong language, preacher!" Well, if it isn't murder, it is negligent homicide to say the least.

In 1848, the physician Ignaz Semmelweis discovered that if the doctors in the Vienna maternity ward would wash their hands, fewer new mothers would die of childbed fever. As a result of this simple change, the mortality rate dropped from 18 percent to one percent. But he was ridiculed and fired from his hospital post. He obtained a similar position in Budapest where he continued to save thousands of lives by the same simple method. Many years later the medical authorities of Europe still ridiculed Semmelweis, even though their mortality rate was 10-15 percent and his was one percent. Why did they oppose this simple natural remedy? The scientific evidence was there, but they were not interested in truth. They were blinded by pride, prejudice, and vested interests. Moses had taught thousands of years earlier that washing was essential to prevent the spread of infections (Lev. 15:13). If medical authorities will resist the Word of God, it is not surprising that they will continue to resist the same truth when it is confirmed with visible scientific evidence.

In the latter part of the 19th century, the French chemist Louis Pasteur discovered that fermentation and some diseases are caused by micro-organisms, today commonly called germs. He met strong opposition from medical authorities. The opposition was unusually intense because he was a chemist, not a physician. He was intruding into areas where others had vested interests. The same is still true today. When a chemist discovers a valuable truth about vitamins or minerals in relation to health, he can expect opposition from medical authorities who do not want any competition.

Again in the late part of the 19th century, the Japanese physician Kanehiro Takaki discovered that the disease of beri-beri was caused by polishing the rice, which removed the B-complex in the outer bran covering. He was ridiculed, but today most of the world has eliminated beri-beri as a result of his discovery of vitamin B_1 in bran.

In 1914, the American physician Joseph Goldberger discovered that the terrible disease of pellagra was a vitamin deficiency disease and that it could be cured by certain natural factors found in liver and yeast. But opposition kept his discovery from being adopted for another quarter of a century. Why? Because the medical establishment was already dedicated to the virus theory of pellagra, and they did not want to admit error. They did not want to change their theories or their practices. So people continued to die. You see, the lives of the patients were not important. The important thing was that the medical authorities must be allowed to rule the doctors without interference from new discoveries. But today pellagra is almost unknown because of Dr. Goldberger's discovery of vitamin B_2.

In about 1928, penicillin was discovered and found to be a powerful antibiotic. However, this substance was not made in man's laboratory. It was a natural substance, grown in a mold, and was ridiculed by the medical powers. They kept it off the market until 1941, when a great flood of war casualties forced this material out into the open in spite of opposition. We may well wonder how many hundreds of thousands of persons died of infection because certain powerful persons in the drug-medical complex did not want competition or interference from this new "quackery."

These are just a few chapters from the disgraceful history of the medical profession. The cases mentioned are public knowledge and may be confirmed by any interested reader merely by referring to any standard reference encyclopedia. The medical world today does not deny that these tragic events did take place. But the usual attitude is that these are errors of the past and could not happen again in our modern "advanced scientific world." Let us see if that is so.

HAS THE WORLD STOPPED OPPOSING GOD?

Has the world progressed and become so enlightened that it no longer opposes the truth of God? The popular belief is that it has. Our school children are routinely taught that man is steadily advancing morally and otherwise and that modern man cannot be guilty of the evils of the past. Nothing could be more false! This delusion of moral advancement is clearly the work of Satan. God's Word does not teach that man will become morally better with the passing of time. Just the opposite! "Evil men and seducers shall wax worse and worse, deceiving and being deceived" (2 Tim. 3:13). If you are not familiar with this Bible truth, then read the 13th chapter of Revelation where you will see that the entire world will one day follow the leadership of Satan, with the exception of a minority group who will repent of their sins and turn to Jesus Christ. The fact that the world will become worse, not better, is universally recognized by all Bible students who take seriously the prophetic portions of Scripture.

At every period of history men can see that their predecessors opposed the truth of God, but they cannot see that they are doing the same thing. The religious leaders in the days of Jesus knew that their fathers had persecuted the prophets of God, but they claimed that they would not be guilty of such a thing (Matt. 23:29-30). They decorated the tombs of the martyred men of God, and were proud that they were more enlightened and would not be guilty of such crimes of the past. Yet at that very time they were persecuting the Son of God! Centuries later the religious powers of Europe looked back on those who persecuted Jesus. They claimed they would not do such a thing, but they burned the followers of Jesus at the stake! Why don't we learn a lesson from this? Man will always oppose God! He will admit that previous generations did this but will deny that he is doing the same thing himself.

Today many of the most powerful men in the religious world do not accept Jesus Christ as the Son of God or as their personal Savior. They even ridicule those who really do trust Jesus, brand them as mentally ill, and seek to hinder the work of Bible-believing Christians. In many parts of the world, true believers are still persecuted unto death, often in the name of religion. No, the world's opposition to God has not stopped. As long as we believe Satan's lie about the "progress" of mankind, we will find it difficult to believe that men will still ridicule the truth of God. But the persecution still goes on, whether we like to realize it or not.

Most of us can probably be convinced that persecution of truth still continues in the religious world, but we may feel that such a thing cannot still happen in the medical world. I ask the question again, "Why do we believe that medical men are more honest and more godly than religious men?" Why is the healing profession thought to be free from the same sinful nature that infects the rest of mankind? The truth is that no part of this evil world has been cured of its evil, not the religious world, not the entertainment world, not the industrial world, and not the medical world.

A growing number of Americans are becoming increasingly convinced that there exists in this country a vast drug-medical-political complex that puts its own financial interests above the welfare of the people. As a student of the Bible, I would believe this to be true even if I saw no other evidence, for it is completely consistent with what the Word of God teaches about the world. If there is religious activity organized against God, political activity organized against God, military activity organized against God, then why not medical activity organized against God? I will present little documentary evidence of this, but for those who wish such documentation, a recommended reading list will be given at the close of this volume. The literature on this subject is abundant. Hundreds of volumes and thousands of pamphlets on the subject are readily available to any reader who will start looking seriously for information.

Even the casual observer can see abundant evidence of an attempt to set up a medical monopoly in this country. In many states other types of healers are systematically destroyed by perfectly legal means. Chiropractors, osteopaths, naturopaths, and other healing arts have been outlawed at many times and in many states. And what is a naturopath? He is simply one who seeks to promote health through nutrition, fasting, exercise, and other natural,

Godgiven methods. But aren't these people quacks? Of course some of them are. But so are some medical doctors. Who is responsible for putting these healers out of business? In many cases it is the state medical association that persuades the legislature to enact such an unfair law.

In this country we have powerful anti-trust laws that seek to prevent one group from destroying competition and getting control of an entire industry. Usually these laws are fairly effective. But in the case of the healing arts, the law has been widely ignored. Those in competition with the medical monopoly have been systematically eliminated in flagrant violation of anti-trust laws and constitutional guarantees of equal protection under the law. Of course, the loophole used to avoid anti-trust laws is to call these outlawed groups quacks. What if General Motors called members of the Chrysler Corporation quacks and had laws passed to put them out of business? What a nice way to destroy the competition! This makes just as much sense as passing laws against chiropractors because the medical competition says they are quacks.

The vitamin scandal in our country is further evidence of a medical monopoly working against God's natural healing. God created vitamins, and He has been using vitamins for centuries to keep people healthy. But in recent years our food processing methods have removed much of the vitamins from our food. As a result, millions of Americans have found that supplementary vitamins help them to feel better and maintain better health. Many of these same persons feel that the American Medical Association, the Food and Drug Administration, and other agencies have waged continual warfare against the use of supplementary vitamins. The methods reportedly used are ridicule, unfair newspaper articles, and oppressive regulation of vitamin dealers. The irony of it all is this: the same FDA that seeks to discourage the public from buying vitamins has permitted the use of hundreds of toxic substances in our food. Think of it! An agency of our government, charged with the responsibility of watching over our health, interferes with our right to buy vitamins—some of them useful against cancer. This same agency allows substances in our food that are universally known to cause cancer! Hard to believe? You had better start reading some of the vast amount of literature now being published on this subject. And you had better believe the Word of God which says, "evil men and seducers shall wax worse and worse" and "the world by wisdom knew not God." And that includes the medical world!

A few years ago a committee of U.S. Senators investigated the slow progress of American medicine. Among other things, they wanted to know what was preventing progress in the field of cancer research. According to a newspaper clipping in my possession, it was the opinion of the committee that organized medicine for fifty years had hindered progress in this area.

For many of my readers, this discovery will come as a crushing shock. Some will find it difficult to believe because they have always assumed that somewhere there was a group of dedicated medical men, completely trustworthy, standing guard over their health. Unfortunately this is not so. Our medical politicians may be princely men, but God's Word warns us not to put our confidence in princes (Ps. 118:8-9). We are to put our confidence only in God.

I am not glad that the world is opposed to God's ways of healing. But since it is true, I am very grateful that I learned about it. If it took cancer to wake me up to this vital bit of knowledge, then "thank you, Lord, for cancer!" My faith is now much less in men, but much greater in our wonderful Lord!

"In every thing give thanks"
(1 Thessalonians 5:18)

I can thank God for cancer, because it led me to understand this surprising biological principle—

PRINCIPLE NO. 6: THE MALIGNANT CELL IS A NORMAL PART OF LIFE

I realize there are two conflicting theories concerning the cause of cancer. I also realize that these two theories lead to two radically different forms of treatment. And the form of treatment one follows can spell the difference of life or death. That is a very serious matter. The theory of cancer origin presented in this chapter is held by many of the worlds' most renowned scientists, but it is still a minority opinion among America's practicing physicians. If this theory is wrong, then it leads to useless therapy, and multitudes of lives might be lost as a result.

But on the other hand, if this theory is true, as I and thousands of others are firmly convinced that it is true, then the more popular theory is false and leads to harmful types of therapy. And again thousands, even millions, of lives are lost because of the error. So you see we cannot be silent. For years now the enemies of this theory have tried everything in their power to silence us, to prevent us from telling what we believe. But we growing thousands of Americans who have come to understand this explanation of cancer have this truth burning in our souls, and we cannot keep silent. Every day one thousand Americans die of cancer, most of them in terrible agony. We believe with all of our heart that many of these could be saved and most of them could have relief from pain if the true nature of cancer was accepted and followed in our medical practice. Fantastic? Then I dare you to read the rest of this book and find out why we believe this so strongly.

The disease called cancer falls in a class all by itself. The malignant cell is different from other body cells. A malignant tumor is a growing mass totally different from the normal surrounding tissues. In other words, a cancer is another form of life, invading your body, competing with normal tissues for nourishment, and destroying other tissues and organs in the process. The big mystery in cancer then is this, "What causes the formation of this special cell, the malignant cell? What is its origin? Where does it come from?" One thousand lives a day in the United States alone depend on the answer to this question. The correct answer leads to adequate prevention, effective treatment, and lives saved. The incorrect answer leads to no prevention, ineffective treatment, untold misery, and lives lost. So dear reader friend, please pay close attention to the following sections. If you understand the truth about the *cause* of cancer, you will then understand the means of *preventing* and *treating* cancer (at least in its early stages). This could save your life and the lives of your loved ones.

THE VIRUS THEORY OF CANCER

For many decades now the most popular theory of cancer origin has been the virus theory. This thesis contends that somehow a virus invasion causes the normal body cells to change to malignant cells. This theory has long been accepted without proof. But in recent years this idea has been strongly challenged, and its supporters are trying desperately to find some scientific evidence to bolster their pet idea. Recent newspaper articles have made much of the fact that researchers have found a virus in a tumor. Big deal! This is supposed to prove that the virus caused the tumor! How absurd can you get? One often finds worms in a rotten log, but this does not indicate that the worms caused the log to be there.

Let us remember that for almost every chronic disease in history, the medical profession has insisted that the cause was some mysterious virus. Now again history is repeating itself. We have another chronic metabolic disease, cancer. Again the experts shout "virus" and spend billions hunting the virus when all the evidence indicates that cancer is yet another disease caused by a nutritional deficiency. Have you forgotten what the evidence is? Practically every tribe of people on earth that eat a completely natural diet, avoiding processed food, are cancer-free or at least have a low incidence of cancer. There is other evidence which we shall discuss later, but this alone is sufficient to practically destroy the virus theory of cancer origin. History has taught us one tragic lesson. When organized medicine adopts the virus theory concerning a chronic disease, they will hold on to this theory long after the disease is proved to be a metabolic problem due to faulty nutrition.

That raises a question: Why? The answer is not hard to find if you believe what the Word of God says about man's depraved nature. Men without Christ are incurably proud and selfish.

The virus theory appeals to natural human pride. According to the virus theory, cancer is so mysterious that the common man is totally helpless to understand it or to do anything about it. He is totally helpless to understand it or to do anything about it. He is totally at the mercy of the professionals. This appeals to their pride, their desire for authority, and their lust for economic advantage. This reminds us of the priests who have told their parishioners not to read the Bible. This was for the professional men of religion only! It was a mystery beyond the common man! Again this suited the lust for gain that was in the hearts of these religious professionals. Isn't it strange how parallel have been the world of religion and the world of medicine?

EVIDENCE AGAINST THE VIRUS THEORY

We have already seen one item of evidence against the idea that cancer is due to a virus. That is the relatively cancer-free life of certain tribes like the Hunzas who eat a totally natural diet. But for the Christian who will do some common sense thinking, there are other serious objections to the virus theory. God created all life. The malignant cell is a living thing, so God must have created it. If the malignant cell is not a normal part of the human life cycle, then this cell comes about by spontaneous generation.

But spontaneous generation is unscriptural and was long ago rejected as scientifically impossible. So-called scientists formerly thought that maggots in spoiled meat were formed there spontaneously. Other small creatures were thought to come about the same way. But now we know life can only come from life. The maggot was seen to be a stage in the life cycle of the fly. So spontaneous generation was centuries ago disproved by science. But now medical science returns to this rejected principle again in its desperate attempt to explain the mystery of cancer. But in spite of this vain attempt, the malignant cell just has to be a normal part of the human life cycle. There are principles of Scripture and also principles of science that demand this.

Another reason for rejecting the virus theory is the tragic consequences of this theory when put into practice. According to this theory, the individual is helpless either to prevent or to treat cancer. All he can do is let the experts try to cut it out, and if that fails try to burn it out, and if that fails try to poison it to death. The results have not been encouraging. In spite of billions spent in cancer research, very little progress has been made. Cancer is on the increase and a rapidly growing number of Americans are becoming skeptical about the value of existing therapies. Too many millions have gone down this familiar trail: surgery, then radiation, then chemotherapy, and—after 15 or 20 thousand dollars are spent—then the grave. The proof of the pudding is in the eating! Our present cancer therapies are a failure! They are a national disgrace! Why? Because the whole system must be based on a false thesis! It is time to abandon the foolish virus theory of cancer and start all over in our research. This theory has failed. Let's try a new theory that will lead to a different form of treatment!

THE TROPHOBLAST THEORY

Before discussing the trophoblast theory of cancer, we must make sure that the reader understands what trophoblast is. So let's just forget about cancer for a moment and talk about trophoblast cells. We are now discussing a well known principle of embryology, something universally recognized by all scientists, something not controversial.

We all know that in conception one male cell unites with one female cell to form one new cell which is the beginning of a new human being. Of course this single cell then divides into two, then four, and so on until a small lump of cells is formed. But what the average layman doesn't think much about is that somewhere down the line different kinds of cells must be formed to accomplish certain specific purposes. There must be bone cells, muscle cells, nerve cells, blood cells, and many others. All of these are different, but all come from the one original cell.

So we can easily see that this one original cell is capable of producing all the different kinds of cells needed for the complete, highly complex human body. At first this small lump of cells is attached to nothing. It merely floats in a fluid environment and absorbs nourishment from that fluid. But soon a crisis situation develops. There is a danger that the new life may fall out of the mother's womb and be lost. But God has a wonderful plan to prevent this. Even the Psalmist David, speaking under the inspiration of the Spirit of God, spoke of the wonders of the embryonic state. "Thou hast covered me in my mother's womb. I will praise thee, for I am fearfully and wonderfully made" (Ps. 139:13-14). Nowhere is this wonder of creation more clearly seen than at this stage of the embryo under discussion. The floating ball of cells must find a way to imbed itself into the inner wall of the uterus, where it can find both secure support and an adequate supply of nourishment. And our all-wise Creator has marvelously provided for this need. The basic cell begins to form a new kind of cell, called the trophoblast. This cell has the unique capacity to eat into surrounding tissue. The trophoblast growth invades and erodes the uterus wall until it is deeply imbedded. The oncoming embryo now can be securely anchored and has a perfect source of nourishment. After about eight weeks the trophoblast cells discontinue their invasion and go no deeper into the uterus wall. No one but

God could have conceived such a wonderful plan. The trophoblast cells perform a miracle. None of us would be alive today if there were no trophoblast cells.

But what does this have to do with cancer? In 1902, Dr. John Beard, Professor of Embryology at Edinburgh, Scotland, discovered that trophoblast cells and cancer cells are identical. The trophoblast cell is malignant and the cancer cell is malignant; both have the power to invade surrounding tissue. At last the mystery of cancer was solved. Cancer cells then do not develop spontaneously because of some strange virus. The cancer cell is a trophoblast, and therefore a normal part of the human life cycle.

Dr. Beard also discovered that a few of these basic cells may become scattered throughout the body. Also these basic human cells have the capacity to form new trophoblast cells under certain conditions. But these trophoblasts are normally kept under control by the enzymes which are manufactured in the pancreas. Enzymes are one of God's natural methods designed to destroy excess trophoblast cells and thus to prevent an abnormal trophoblast growth in the body. Dr. Beard demonstrated that cancer could not take place where there was a sufficient supply of these pancreatic enzymes. And pancreatic deficiency is often the result of metabolic imbalance related to poor nutrition.

The reader may wonder why the medical world did not immediately seize this opportunity to stop this dreadful disease. Have you forgotten the history of the medical profession? Why did they wait 260 years to stop scurvy after the cure was known? Why did they wait 30 years to stop pellagra after the cure was known? The medical profession is always highly resistant to new discoveries, especially if they involve a simple, natural solution for a terrible disease. This is inexcusable, of course, but it is understandable. To accept this new idea would involve discarding time honored text books. Entire medical libraries would become useless. Courses which have been taught for years in medical schools would have to be abandoned or rewritten. Billions of dollars worth of medical equipment would become obsolete. Medical schools would have to admit that their teachings were harmful. Physicians who were secure in their practice would be upset. They would have to start over and become students again. And then there would be the families of the patients who died because of the earlier useless therapies. They may become angry. The physician is in a serious predicament. This new idea threatens his position of great respect in the community and it also threatens his economic security.

So what happened to Dr. Beard's wonderful discovery? His writings were filed away in medical archives and rejected as being too revolutionary to be put into practical use. History had repeated itself. The reader must realize that there are two stages in solving any serious chronic disease. The first stage is the scientific one. A scientific explanation of the disease must be found, and this is usually the easiest part. The second stage is much harder for it involves the overcoming of economic and political resistance to the new discovery. The scientific conquest of cancer began in 1902. After more than seventy years the political battle has not yet been won. If the reader finds it difficult to believe that organized medicine would resist the truth that long, then just remember that it resisted the vitamin C treatment for scurvy for 260 years!

If the reader is to understand how to protect himself from cancer, he must realize this truth. The malignant cell is a normal part of the life cycle. God made the malignant cell for a purpose. The Psalmist wrote:

> Thine eyes did see my substance, yet being unperfect; and in thy book all my members were written, which in continuance were fashioned, when as yet there was none of them. (Ps. 139:16)

God new every part of you. He knew every kind of cell that played a part in the formation of your body. He knew all about the trophoblast cell, and in His goodness and wisdom He made a way for it to be kept under control. Cancer then is an improper multiplication of trophoblast cells, at the wrong place, at the wrong time. Since God planned a way to prevent this, such a growth is due to man's failure to cooperate with God's laws of health, particularly in the matter of nutrition.

EVIDENCE FOR THE TROPHOBLAST THEORY

If the traditional virus theory is true, then man can do nothing about cancer but cut it, burn it, poison it. On the other hand, if the trophoblast theory is true, then cancer can be prevented by proper nutrition and can be controlled by natural means, at least in the early stages. No doubt many will read these lines whose lives will hinge on making the right decision here. With so much at stake, I don't blame anyone for being slow to accept the trophoblast theory. Each reader should have the freedom to choose for himself. No one else should decide for you. The evidence I am about to give here is given in the interest of fairness. The evidence for the virus theory (if any) has been abundantly represented. The newspapers and other mass media have promoted this theory for decades. But most Americans have not had the opportunity to look at the other side of the story. I believe every human being has a right to consider the evidence for the trophoblast theory so that he may decide for himself which course he will take, for cancer is an ever present threat to every one of us. I suggest here several items of evidence, to which the reader should give serious consideration. I know from experience that most laymen (in the medical sense) who are reverent Christians will find the trophoblast theory easy to accept. The more skeptical reader, with scientific background, will no doubt say that the proof is not absolute. Perhaps so, but at least you can see that the theory rests on pretty sound footing and should be thoroughly investigated.

The Testimony of Theology. The trophoblast theory is consistent with the Biblical teachings about God. God created all things. God is wise and good. It is just like God to provide natural means to keep the malignant trophoblast cell under control.

The Testimony of Biology. The body has a wonderful system of balances. For example, we cannot live without salt, yet the body has ways of eliminating excess salt. The same is true of many chemical elements. The body must not have too much or too little, so God has provided in nature various methods to maintain the balance. The same is true of the white blood cells and red blood cells. We must not have too few or too many. The body has ways to control this. So why should we think it strange that the malignant cell is normally kept in balance by natural body mechanisms?

The Testimony of History. For centuries every time someone discovers a natural, God-given cure for a terrible disease, powerful and cruel opposition rises up to oppose it. Since the cure is planned by God, we must conclude that this violent and cruel opposition comes from Satan. Of course Satan uses men who usually do not know that Satan is using them. It has been often said that you can know a man by his enemies. You can also know a principle by its enemies. When violent and unreasonable opposition is directed against a simple natural solution to a terrible disease, then the lesson of history would suggest that this unreasonable opposition must be from the devil, and the natural remedy must be of God. History then would warn us to seriously consider the trophoblast theory of cancer and the natural preventions that are corollaries to this theory.

The Testimony of Cytology. Scientists in different parts of the world have reported that they have found 250 ways in which the trophoblast cell and the cancer cell are alike. They also report that they have found no way in which they differ. Cancer researchers in this country, already devoted to the virus theory, do not try to refute this evidence. They just close their eyes, ignore the evidence, and continue to spend the huge cancer research grants from the government (which of course comes from your pockets and mine as taxpayers). Remember this principle: It is more profitable to hunt for a cancer cure than it is to find one!

The Testimony of Embryology. What causes the trophoblast to stop growing in the mother's womb during pregnancy? Why doesn't this placenta (really a cancer) keep growing until it destroys both mother and child? Here again we see the wisdom and goodness of Almighty God. After eight weeks of development, the baby's pancreas begins to function, pouring out the enzyme trypsin into the bloodstream. This, added to the mother's trypsin, is sufficient to stop further trophoblast activity. This well known fact further supports the entire theory.

The Testimony of Pathology. Cancer can strike any part of the body, but there is one large area of the body that is almost totally free of this disease. This is the upper intestine, or small intestine. Why is this part of the body so well protected? Only the trophoblast theory explains this phenomenon. The pancreas discharges its secretions through a duct, which opens into the digestive tract just below the stomach at the upper end of the intestines. Cancer of the stomach is common, but cancer at the upper end of the intestine is almost unknown. Why? The heavy concentration of trypsin at this point makes cancer almost impossible. But the further down we go into the intestinal tract, the higher is the incidence of cancer. Cancer is quite common in the lower intestine (colon) and extremely frequent in the sigmoid and rectal area because the trypsin becomes more diluted as it passes downward through the alimentary canal and thus becomes less effective. These are recognized facts, but only the trophoblast theory explains why.

The Testimony of Medical Experience. While the majority of physicians in this country has not seriously considered the trophoblast theory and its practical implications, twenty-four major foreign nations are making good progress against cancer, based on this theory. Some of the world's foremost cancer authorities base much of their treatment on the principle of pancreatic enzymes, which is a part of the trophoblast theory. Hundreds of cancer patients, who have been given up to die by orthodox physicians in this country, travel to clinics in other countries where they receive enzyme therapy or nutritional therapy, both based on the trophoblast theory. Even though most of these patients are near death when they begin the new therapy, nevertheless many of them are wonderfully helped. Another victory for the trophoblast theory!

The Testimony of Common Experience. Tens of thousands of cancer patients around the world will testify to objective improvement after adding supplementary pancreatic enzymes to their nutritional program. This writer personally knows a famous biochemist who has taught in a number of America's medical schools. Thirty years ago a large tumor was discovered on his colon. Immediate surgery was absolutely necessary, he was told. But he did not have the surgery. For thirty years he has kept the tumor under control, using only enzyme therapy.

Today at the age of 80 he is still active and in surprisingly good health. While surgery is often useless to the cancer patient, there are times when it helps. For example, a surgeon may remove a large tumor, neat and clean. Soon thereafter, a smaller tumor in the patient disappears. Why? Only the trophoblast theory gives an answer. The patient did not have sufficient enzymes to fight both tumors. But with the big one gone, the natural enzymes dissolve the remaining small one. Chalk up another victory for the trophoblast theory! I believe these items of evidence deserve your most serious consideration. Don't you believe now that God is in the cancer-fighting business?

To conclude this chapter, let us summarize the two prevailing theories of cancer origin and note the conclusions that logically follow in each case.

The Virus Theory	The Trophoblast Theory
The cancer cell *is not* a normal part of the human life cycle.	The cancer cell *is* a normal part of the human life cycle.
The cancer cell is formed when a virus changes a normal body cell into an abnormal malignant cell.	The cancer cell is the same as the common trophoblast cell and is therefore perfectly normal.

Since the cancer cell is not a normal part of the body, the body is not equipped with any means to keep it under control.	Since the cancer cell is a normal part of the body, the body has normal anti-cancer defenses built into it by nature.
Since the cancer cell is not a normal part of the body or the total environment, there is nothing in our environment designed to fight the cancer cell.	Since the cancer cell is a normal part of nature, there are natural substances in our food supply that oppose excessive multiplication of these cancer cells. This is part of the balance of nature.
Since the cancer cell was not planned by God, God did not design any cancer-fighting mechanisms in nature.	Since the cancer cell was created by God, He was wise enough and good enough to plan natural defenses against it in our bodies and in our food supply.
God *does not* regularly fight cancer by natural means.	God *does* regularly fight cancer by natural means.
Since God has no regular means of controlling the malignant cell, man is helpless and has	Since God has a regular means of controlling the malignant cell, it is possible to cooperate with His methods and

no way to prevent cancer.

Since God has no regular means of fighting cancer, only medical science can fight cancer. The cancer patient is helpless. He can do nothing for himself. He is totally dependent on the professionals. His only hope is in surgery, radiation, chemotherapy, etc.

Since there are no cancer-fighting substances in nature, those who seek to prevent or control cancer by natural means are "quacks" and should be put in jail—so their enemies teach.

thus to prevent cancer.

Since God has natural means of controlling cancer, the cancer patient can do much to help himself especially if he does not wait too long. The patient and his family are morally obligated to learn God's methods and to cooperate with them.

Since God did put cancer-fighting substances in nature, those who seek to fight cancer by these natural means are cooperating with Almighty God. They are the greatest of all cancer researchers. They are extremely unselfish, dedicated, and courageous to proceed with this valuable research in the face of such cruel opposition. They deserve to be honored among the greatest heroes of our land.

IT CERTAINLY MAKES A LOT OF DIFFERENCE WHICH ONE OF THESE THEORIES YOU BELIEVE!

One of the greatest discoveries of my entire lifetime is the fact that the cancer cell is a natural part of life. This removes the mystery. This sheds an entirely different light on the problem. This is the foundation for understanding and combating cancer. This opens up a whole new world of cancer prevention and cancer treatment. I am thrilled beyond measure at this discovery. I probably would have never learned this if I had not had cancer myself. Then I could not have helped others understand it. So that's why I thank God for cancer.

"In every thing give thanks"
(1 Thessalonians 5:18)

I can thank God for cancer, because it led me to understand this wonderful principle of creation—

PRINCIPLE NO. 7: GOD PROVIDES FOR CANCER CONTROL IN NATURE

Do you find it difficult to believe that nature has its own powerful and efficient methods of combating the malignant cell? Why should this be surprising? Our all-wise Creator put vitamin C in our environment to prevent scurvy. He provided vitamin B_2 to prevent pellagra, and this list of known preventatives could go on and on. And so we really ought to *expect* that He also placed anti-cancer materials in our natural environment. All it takes to arrive at such a conclusion is a deep respect for God and some logical thinking. Fortunately we now also have much supporting evidence.

In recent years man has learned to appreciate the principle of balance in nature. In every location, plants, animals, and insects live in a balanced ecological system. No species can overpopulate because other forms of life prevent it. The same is true within the human body. The red blood cells, white blood cells, trophoblast cells, and other biological and chemical factors keep each other in balance. But man often upsets the balance of nature. Some islands have been totally ruined because man destroyed one form of life, and thus upset the balance of nature. The balance of the body can also be upset. For example, we must have *some* white blood cells, but if they become too numerous, they may become a dangerous threat to the red blood cells. Since this is a well known fact, why should it surprise us to learn that malignant cells (trophoblasts) have a similar pattern? We need some of them, but if they become too numerous, we may be in trouble. Nature's way of preventing cancer then is to maintain the proper balance of body metabolism.

What causes the trophoblast cells to multiply and become so numerous as to cause a tumor? There is overwhelming evidence that this is caused by the removal of anti-cancer materials from our food supply. There are many cancer-resistant peoples in the world, and the cancer fighting substances in their diet are known to science. But these same people become cancer-prone when they adopt the diet of Western man. Details explaining how these anti-trophoblastic substances have been removed from our diet will be given later. At this point, the reader should understand that the trophoblast goes out of control because of faulty nutrition, and it can often be brought back under control by adequate nutrition.

NATURE PREVENTS AND CONTROLS, BUT DON'T EXPECT A CURE

The enemies of nutritional cancer control are skilled in the art of slander. They are constantly ridiculing these "foolish natural cancer cures." This is most interesting! I have read many of the books on nutritional therapy, have attended several conventions dealing with these principles, and have heard many physicians lecture on the subject, but not once have I heard one of them claim to cure cancer. They only speak of prevention and control. This is powerful evidence that such men are not quacks as their enemies claim. One of the identifying marks of a quack is the boastful and dogmatic claims he makes concerning cures. Nutritional scientists are the most cautious men I have known. They realize the vast complexity of body chemistry. They realize that there are many variables—some of them still unknown—in any case of recovery. And so, characteristically, they do not make wild claims of an absolute cure. But they do know from worldwide evidence that cancer can be prevented by proper nutrition. And they also know from clinical experience that it can often be brought under control by natural means, even after it has progressed considerably.

Why is it not wise to speak of curing cancer? Cancer is a very special disease; it destroys surrounding tissues and even vital organs. Let's look at a comparison. If a man is shot with a bullet, and the bullet damaged a vital organ, can he be cured? Perhaps not. Merely removing the bullet certainly would not be a cure. He could still die from the damage. Likewise if a cancer is completely destroyed by natural means, this is not necessarily a cure. The patient can still die because of the damaged organ. And because trophoblast cells can always grow out of control again, the cancer patient is wise to never consider himself cured. He should think in terms of keeping the malignancy under control. And if he is wise, this will mean a lifetime of cautious living. No doubt there are cases where the cure is complete, but the patient can never be sure of this. You see, God did not plan for us to get cancer and then cure it. He obviously intended for us to prevent it. So let's cooperate with God and think in terms of prevention and control!

HOW CAN WE KNOW ABOUT CANCER-PREVENTING SUBSTANCES?

Perhaps some of my readers are still wondering, "If there are anti-cancer materials in our natural environment, why doesn't the scientific world universally accept this fact?" I have already given some of the reasons, and shall give additional reasons later in this book. But first we need to understand the different sources of knowledge and belief. We can distinguish four such sources.

Revelation. The Bible, the revealed Word of God, is the highest source of knowledge. Of course the Scriptures do not deal at length with specific health information because it is primarily a book of *spiritual* truth. However it does establish certain principles and it does make an occasional reference that sheds light on our health problems. We will continue to mention such references throughout this work.

Laboratory Science. This refers to experiments conducted under carefully controlled conditions, where precise measurements are made and careful records kept. This of course is a very valuable source of knowledge, but it does have its limitations. As we have shown before, and shall show again, man's greed and selfish heart can even pervert the results of so-called scientific research. Laboratory science has contributed much to our knowledge of health, but it is by no means the *exclusive* source of such knowledge, as we shall see.

Empirical Knowledge. This refers to information gained by common people over a long period of time as they observe what happens. For example, thousands of years ago, farmers discovered that fertilizer—decaying organic matter—buried near the roots of plants would cause greater growth and more fruit. They did not know why this worked. It had not been proven in careful scientific experiments. But it worked! Now suppose that some "scientist" had come along and tried to persuade them that this procedure was not dependable because its cause had not been confirmed by "science." The farmer would never accept such arguments, science or no science. You see, we can know from long experience that some things are true, even though the "scientific experts" have not found the reason and they may say that it is not confirmed.

This is the principle behind folk medicine. While some ideas of folk medicine may be erroneous, much of it is wonderfully true because it has been confirmed by centuries of observation. Folk medicine can be highly accurate in many cases, and is often decades or centuries ahead of so-called medical science, as we shall soon see.

Superstition. The fourth and least valuable

source of knowledge or belief is legend or superstition. It is important to notice the vast difference in folk medicine and superstition. Folk medicine is based on long observed facts, while superstition often persists in flagrant opposition to observed facts. For example, many people in India superstitiously believe that bathing in the Ganges River will heal their diseases. But the river is filled with pollution, sewage, and infections. Careful observation would no doubt reveal that in most cases the patient is worse rather than better after such a bath. But the *superstition persists in spite of evidence to the contrary.*

Unscientific superstition is more likely to occur in pagan lands where the people do not have the light of the gospel and are subject to the deception of Satan. On the other hand, folk medicine is more likely to develop in lands with a Christian background, where the people have a respect for God and for natural law, and where they carefully observe the things of nature to see what these laws are.

There is a very good reason why I am stressing this difference between folk medicine and superstition. Many anti-cancer substances have been discovered through centuries of observation. Call it folk medicine if you wish, because in some cases it is not known *how* the materials fight cancer. But the enemies of such natural healing try to prejudice the public against these remedies by calling them "superstition." But this is a lie! If the idea of natural healing persisted for centuries in spite of failure, this would be superstition. But the belief in natural anti-cancer substances is based on centuries of observing the *successes*. This is quite another matter. Many things may be known by the careful observer, even though the "scientific experts" do not yet understand it. So please remember that nutritional prevention of cancer is not based on legend or superstition, but rather on centuries of observation.

SOME POSSIBLE ANTI-CANCER SUBSTANCES IN NATURE

As we have already mentioned, there seem to be many natural anti-cancer materials in nature's food supply. Some of them are more plentiful in certain parts of the world, but apparently no part of the world is completely without them. I will not go into much detail in this book, because that is not my purpose. The literature on this subject is already abundant, and I have no desire to repeat what has already been written. My purpose is to give hope to the cancer patient, to encourage him to believe that God is at work in this field, and to encourage him to read the available literature and to learn to care for his health. So my discussion of anti-cancer substances will be merely a brief summary, without attempting any proof.

Enzymes. An enzyme is an organic catalyst. A

catalyst is a chemical substance that causes other chemicals to react but is not changed itself. A tiny quantity of an enzyme can cause a chemical process involving very large quantities of material, and the enzyme is not worn out or used up in the process. So we might say that an enzyme is God's miracle drug. Over seven hundred different enzymes are known to be at work in the human body, all of them performing chemical wonders that make man's most complex chemical plants look simple by comparison. Some of these play a part in protecting the body against the malignant cell. The enzymes trypsin and chymotrypsin, secreted by the pancreas, play a powerful role in destroying excess trophoblasts. Other enzymes from the food supply are vitally important in many aspects of health, including cancer prevention. All growing plants are abundantly rich in enzymes. In fact, it is the enzymes that cause the wonders of plant growth. Unfortunately, most enzymes are destroyed by heat, and that explains why raw fruits and vegetables are so important to general health and cancer prevention.

Vitamins. A vitamin is not some childish fad as some have imagined. The word *vitamin* is from the Latin word *vita,* meaning *life.* Nutritional research has shown that all the principal vitamins play a part in cancer prevention. For example, one group of mice is fed an ideal diet, and a second group is fed the same diet except with a vitamin A deficiency. The group deprived of vitamin A has far more cancers; the same experiment with other vitamins gives similar results. Natural foods contain abundant vitamins, but our modern food-processing methods remove most of them from our diet. No *vita*mins, no life.

Minerals. The body must have relatively large quantities of certain mineral elements, such as calcium, phosphorus, and iron. But smaller quantities of many other minerals are necessary. These are sometimes called *trace minerals,* because only a trace is needed. In some cases even this tiny trace is missing from the diet, with disastrous results. Some authorities now suspect that the body must have at least a trace of every element in our environment, over a hundred of which are now known. This is consistent with the Biblical teaching that man is made from earth substance.

The vital importance of trace minerals can be seen from the fact that a large and complex enzyme molecule may require one tiny atom of a specific mineral element. This one enzyme molecule can work almost indefinitely, catalyzing a complex chemical reaction, which over a period of time could involve a sizable mass of material. One atom of the right mineral at the right time could have enormous consequences. Both minerals and vitamins are important because they are often parts of complex enzyme systems.

Proteins. The word protein is from the Greek word *protos,* meaning *first.* The protein is first in importance of all nutrients. Every organ, every tissue, and nearly every cell in the body is composed mostly of protein. The blood, the glandular secretions, and most body fluids are largely protein. If the intake of protein is inadequate, the muscles will be consumed to supply this need. Too much protein or too little are both bad for the cancer patient. If there is insufficient protein in the diet, the body will be unable to manufacture enzymes, for they are protein substances. If there is too much protein in the diet, then enzymes that should be digesting cancer cells will be busy digesting protein instead. So a steady diet of a moderate amount of daily protein is best.

Grapes. For centuries there has been a firm belief among millions of earth's population that the grape is a powerful force against cancer. The reasons for this are not fully known, but it has been observed that those who live and work all their life in grape vineyards rarely have cancer. There are several possible reasons for this. The grape ranks very high in protein content. It is rich in minerals, vitamins, and enzymes. It is high in potassium, and some cancer researchers report that many cancer patients are low in potassium. The grape also is acid-forming, and an acid colon is important to cancer resistance in that area.

Bible students who believe in the "grape

cure" have often pointed out that the grape is prominent in Biblical symbolism, and that the juice of the grape is always symbolic of the blood of Jesus Christ that cleanses us from sin. Could there be a connection here? Johanna Brandt is the author of the book, *The Grape Cure*, which has had a wide distribution in many lands. It is my opinion that the word *control* would be better than *cure* here. Also it is unlikely that every malignancy could be brought under control by grapes alone. Every cancer patient is an individual with his own body chemistry and his own particular metabolic problems. Not all respond equally to the same treatment. However, empirical evidence does indicate that the grape has made a great contribution to health in general and to cancer prevention in particular.

Chaparral. Many Indian tribes have long believed that the desert plant chaparral would cure cancer. There is a case on record of an Indian who was dismissed as hopelessly incurable by the university hospital in a Western state. He went to an Indian healer for chaparral treatment and returned to the hospital to amaze the doctors by his apparent cure. I have seen a report of later chaparral research by this same hospital. They apparently experimented with only hopelessly terminal patients and used no treatment other than chaparral. Only fourteen percent of the patients showed improvement, and the researchers felt that this evidence was inconclusive. Can you imagine that? Fourteen percent improved on one plant alone! We wonder how many would have improved if an effort had been made to balance the entire body metabolism, rather than just adding one valuable substance. Unfortunately there seems to be insufficient knowledge as to *how* chaparral works. No doubt it supplies valuable minerals, vitamins, and enzymes. It also aids oxygenation of the blood. But it probably would not work equally well on all patients because each person has different nutritional shortages.

Yogurt. Yogurt is natural to Bible lands and has been a common food and disease fighter there for thousands of years. In the Middle East and the Balkan States, there is widespread belief that yogurt contributes to long life and vitality and that it discourages cancer, especially in the digestive tract. For decades, natural food advocates have claimed this; organized medicine has denied it with equal insistence. Recently a research team in an American university completed a ten-year study of mice on a yogurt diet. They reported a vastly lower percentage of intestinal cancer in the mice that ate the yogurt compared to the control group. This research was done by "orthodox" medical scientists. Time and time again the "orthodox" physicians have had to eat their words and admit they were wrong and the natural food advocates—or "health nuts"—were right after all! One way that yogurt may combat intestinal cancer may be in the formation of vitamin B-complex. The active organism in yogurt is the beneficial bacteria, *Lactobacillus acidophilus.* This friendly little fellow thrives in a healthy intestinal tract, and manufactures many factors of the B-complex. Several B-complex factors play a part in combating cancer. Yogurt was very common in Bible times. Many times the words *milk* or *cheese* in our English translations actually should be *yogurt.*

The Acid-Alkaline Balance. Acids and alkalis are relatively simple compounds, extremely simple in comparison to some of the vast and complex protein substances that are active in the human body. Man is always searching for sophisticated and difficult solutions to his problems, and often overlooks the simple things. Even the Word of God warns of those who despise small things. Some biochemists, in their search for great things, may have overlooked the enormous importance of the acid-alkali balance of body fluids. Of course acids and alkalis are opposites and they neutralize each other. The degree of acid or alkali strength is measured in a scale which chemists call pH. The pH value of pure water is 7, which is considered neutral. A pH value greater than 7 is alkaline; a pH below 7 is acid. As mentioned before, the colon must be acid if it is to remain healthy. The reason is that the *Lactobacillus acidophilus* can live only in an acid medium. The name *acidophilus* means *acid-loving.* If the colon becomes alkaline, the helpful *acidophilus* bacteria die, and harmful bacteria are able to take over in the alkaline environment. The divinely planned chemical factories in the colon are destroyed and no more B-complex is manufactured. The harmful bacteria causes gas, diarrhea, and other intestinal problems. If this is prolonged over a considerable period of time, the result can be chronic colitis, ulcerative colitis, with polyps developing and then malignancy. Remember that colon cancer develops best in an unhealthy colon, and sufficient hydrochloric acid helps to promote colon health.

There is a growing realization that large number of Americans are deficient in hydrochloric acid, which is manufactured in the stomach. This deficiency is especially likely to occur in older persons. This writer knows of one prominent medical laboratory that does blood serum analyses on large numbers of persons. They report that most cancer patients they have studied are low in hydrochloric acid. This is not surprising if we remember how the digestive system works. The moment food is swallowed, it comes under the influence of the gastric juices of the stomach, the chief ingredient of which is hydrochloric acid. It is obvious then that God intended for all nutrition to begin in an acid medium. Proteins are broken down by hydrochloric acid. Such vital minerals as clacium, potassium, and iron can best be assimilated in an acid medium. Many trace minerals cannot be absorbed unless sufficient acid is present. Some enzymes are totally inactive until they come into contact with acid. For this reason some nutritional scientists are saying that "everything begins with acid." This seems to be true. The lowly, simple, and inexpensive hydrochloric acid molecule is apparently then the very foundation of highly complex human metabolism. Truly this is the day of small things!

Now let's come to the practical significance of all this. If the contents of the stomach become either too acid or too alkaline, the symptoms are about the same. The victim may have a bloating, sour stomach, indigestion, etc. Now wouldn't common sense tell you that there is just as much chance for one to have too little acid as too much? And yet our culture has developed the "acid stomach" theory. Thanks to misleading advertising, every person who has stomach distress is told that this is caused by excess stomach acid and that he should correct it by purchasing a certain brand of alkalizer. Now think of the enormous consequences! At least half of these people already have too little acid, or too much alkali which means the same thing. But he goes to the drug store and consumes more alkali, which is to him a deadly poison! But he may get a bit of temporary relief due to some peppermint or other flavoring in the concoction. He does not know that he has made his condition worse! And he may be setting the stage for the eventual development of intestinal cancer, not to mention a host of other lesser ailments. No person should consume antacids or alkalizers unless he has had his pH tested and knows that he needs it. Some physicians recommend antacids merely from symptoms, without testing. Yet the patient may already be suffering from acid deficiency. One may get a fair idea of his bodily pH situation by testing the urine with pH paper that is available in most drug stores and health food stores. Some physicians recommend that the pH of the urine should be 6 or lower, some say 5 or lower, and some recommend as low as 4.5. Professional guidance would be best here. My experience has been that when the pH goes above 5.5, colon problems soon develop. Many others report a similar situation. The pH is lowered by taking hydrochloric acid tablets or capsules which may be purchased at any drug store or health food store.

Some may wonder *why* so many people in our society suffer from acid deficiency. One simple explanation is our enormously high carbohydrate consumption. As a nation we have gone all out for convenience foods which are mostly carbohydrate. And carbohydrates form alkalis when digested. And so the disgracefully high carbohydrate intake of the American people is probably another indirect contributor to our rising cancer problem.

Food Fiber. For many decades most of the food fiber has been removed from the American diet. The outer bran has been removed from our cereal grains. Our fruits and vegetables are cooked and overcooked until much of the cellulose fiber is destroyed. The result has been a bland diet, a soft gooey mess that our intestines were not designed to handle. The peristaltic motions of the intestines are designed to push forward a semi-solid mass that has considerable cohesion. But the soft pasty mixture resulting from a fiberless diet does not move forward properly. Excess pressure and ballooning of the intestine can result. Bulging pockets may form creating a condition known as diverticulosis. Waste matter may collect in these pockets and decay. One intestinal problem leads to another. The standard procedure for decades has been to put the patient on a bland diet that would not irritate the damaged colon. But it was a fiberless diet that caused the problem in the first place. Thank God for the British and South African scientists that discovered this fact. The new treatment for this condition is now to add food fiber to the diet, usually in the form of bran. The results are very encouraging. Chalk up another victory for the "health food nuts." They have been telling us for decades that the removal of bran from our diet would lead to disastrous results. Once more the "orthodox scientists" discovered that they had been wrong and the natural food advocates had been right all the time.

Indirectly this problem is related to the cancer problem. A great amount of cancer begins in the colon and then spreads to other organs. So the eating of whole grain cereals, raw fruits and vegetables, and other natural foods containing sufficient fiber should promote healthy colons and thus reduce the incidence of cancer in our society. It has been noticed that the diet of rural Africans contains much fiber, and these people are remarkably free from the many intestinal problems that plague the western man. You just can't beat God's way of eating, can you?

Fasting. Fasting was a common practice in Bible times. Nowhere is fasting commanded, but everywhere that it is mentioned it seems to be approved. People in Bible lands fasted for physical reasons and also for spiritual reasons. Much literature is available today outlining methods and benefits of this ancient practice. Nearly all physicians and scientists agree on one thing, and that is that Americans are bringing on themselves a host of ailments by overeating. It logically follows then that fasting would prevent or reverse some of these conditions. Much has been written on the probable relationship between overeating and cancer. The theory of fasting as an anti-cancer practice is very simple and logical. The same enzymes that digest food proteins also have a tendency to digest cancer cells. So when the digestive tract is completely empty, these enzymes have no food protein on which to work and can concentrate on digesting cysts, polyps, or tumors. Many experimenters have shown that in practice this often takes place. No doubt the Lord had excellent reasons for encouraging this practice among His ancient people.

The Bitter Almond. Four thousand years ago the Chinese learned that tumors could be successfully treated with bitter almonds. Little did they realize that they were beginning a therapy that would rock the medical world! They did not know what it was in the almond that was so helpful to cancer control, but today top scientists in many nations know exactly what it is and exactly how it works chemically. Other peoples in other parts of the world came to the same conclusion, even without any knowledge of the Chinese discoveries. Folk medicine in several lands has observed that those who work in the bitter almond orchards and ingest large quantities of this nut almost never have cancer. Bible students have found it interesting to note that the almond is a symbol of the resurrection of Jesus Christ (Num. 17:8). Could this be significant? We must keep in mind that the common sweet almond of our country has been tampered with by man and is not the same as the original bitter almond that God made in the first place. Our common almond is a valuable food. It does contain some excellent proteins, vitamins, minerals, and enzymes. But it contains little of the specific anti-cancer agent vitamin B-17 found in the bitter almond.

I have listed here a few of the foods that are believed by many to play a part in the prevention and control of malignancy. These beliefs vary from one location to another, depending of course on what foods are available. But few parts of the world seem to be free of these convictions that are based on long local experience. Much of this is folk medicine, but much of it is beginning to find confirmation in the laboratory. These beliefs, though varying according to location, do not by any means contradict each other. In fact they complement each other in a most wonderful way. As a Christian it would be difficult for me to believe that God placed *only one* cancer-fighting food in the world. It is just like our wonderful Lord to place many such materials in our environment so that all peoples around the world would have access to some of them. All of these substances have considerable empirical evidence to support them. Perhaps not all of them are equal. And there is no evidence that any one of them would prevent cancer in everybody. In most cases the reason for the benefit, if any, is not known. Yet the person interested in combating malignancy should not overlook any of these possibilities. We can sincerely hope that later experience and research will shed more light on these and other natural cancer therapies. Let us turn now to the substance that is rapidly gaining the reputation as nature's most powerful and most specific anti-cancer material.

VITAMIN B-17, NATURE'S CHEMOTHERAPY

The substance we are about to discuss now is in a class all by itself. Its chemical structure and chemical properties are well known to scientists around the world. The exact way it performs chemically in the malignant cell is well known. The theory of its performance is consistent with all known principles of chemistry, and in practice it has been found to work exactly as theory indicates it should. So we are not now dealing with legend, superstition, or folk medicine. We are now discussing pure laboratory science, confirmed by clinical experience.

In order to better understand this specific anti-cancer substance in nature, we need to know something of its history. Beginning about 1840, it was listed for many years in all standard reference books on pharmacology. It was known as *amygdalin*. The name comes from a Greek word meaning *almond* because the substance was first discovered in the bitter almond. Amygdalin was commonly used to treat a variety of ailments including asthma, allergies, arthritis, and high blood pressure. It is still used today for these purposes, often with very good results. Unfortunately this substance has been ignored in pharmacology, and the reason is quite simple. Our society is getting away from

God and away from nature. Medical practitioners find powerful, toxic, manmade chemicals more exciting than simple herbs or natural substances. And so natural materials have gradually been eliminated from the list to make room for the almost endless supply of new products coming from the drug factories. Consequently, today only a few physicians know about the benefits of amygdalin, now commonly known as vitamin B-17.

In 1952, Ernst Krebs, a San Francisco biochemist, made a discovery that may well prove to be the greatest medical discovery of all time. Knowing the chemistry of the cancer cell and the chemical properties of amygdalin, he noticed that in theory the amygdalin should release poisonous cyanide at the cancer cell but not at other cells. Experiments confirmed the theory, for that is exactly what happened. At last he had discovered the long-sought-for anticancer material of nature. The Creator had not left the cancer cell free to run amuck without opposition. He had planned in nature a natural enemy of the malignant cell. Of course we now understand why the Chinese long ago were successful in treating tumors with an extract of bitter almonds. Dr. Krebs learned how to purify amygdalin and developed a purified product as anti-cancer drug under the name *Laetrile*.

How does it work? Its success depends on the marvels of enzymes. These enzymes are the only substance known that have the power to split the amygdalin molecule and release the poisonous cyanide that is locked up in the molecule.* The enzymes are found in significant quantities in only one place, the malignant cells of humans and animals. This wonder of nature could not be a coincidence. This had to be planned by an intelligent Creator. This is the handiwork of God! The common body cells (somatic cells) are in no danger from the cyanide because they do not contain the enzyme beta-glucosidase and therefore no cyanide is formed at the somatic cells. But our wonderful Lord does not stop with one form of protection. He protects the body cells by yet another method. The enzyme rhodenase has the power to instantly convert poisonous cyanide into a substance that is harmless, yes, even nourishing to somatic cells. And rhodenase is found in the somatic cell, not the malignant cell. So even if a small quantity of cyanide released at the cancer cell should spill over onto a body cell, the enzyme rhodenase would immediately convert it before any harm could take place. So it is quite plain that God in nature designed a wonderful and intricate plan to kill off excess trophoblasts and to prevent the development of malignant tumors. This is God's chemotherapy! How much better off we would be if "orthodox" medical research had sought for God's chemotherapy instead of manufacturing the deadly experimental chemicals that today are distributed under the label of chemotherapy.

Where is amygdalin found? The bitter almond is by no means the only source. It is found in over 1200 edible plants, and no part of the world is without a natural supply of amygdalin. The richest known source is found in the seeds of such fruits as the apricot, peach, plum, cherry, apple, etc. Many grasses are rich in amygdalin, as are the outer bran coatings of some grains. All animals in their natural habitat have adequate supplies of amygdalin, and they have no cancer. Animals contact cancer only when man interferes with their natural diet. God taught all the animals how to eat to prevent cancer. Only man deliberately violates God's nutritional plan. This is not surprising when we realize that only men are sinners and rebels against God; animals are not. It is interesting to note that the apricot seed is now considered the richest source of this life-sustaining food factor, and Biblical geographers tell us the apricot is one of the most plentiful fruits in the region of the ancient Garden of Eden!

Why is it that we no longer have adequate supplies of the anti-cancer vitamin B-17 in our diet? This is another disastrous result of food processing and other man-made nutritional changes. For example, millet, which is rich in B-17, was once the common grain in our land. Now it has been replaced by wheat which contains no B-17. Other grains that contain B-17 in the outer bran are now polished and the anti-cancer vitamin is lost to human nutrition.

Sorghum cane, rich in B-17, was once America's principal source of sweeteners. Now it has been replaced by sugar cane which is practically devoid of B-17. Native peaches and other fruits once contained B-17 in the fleshy part of the fruit, but our modern cultivated fruit no longer contains B-17 except in the seed. Why? Man wanted to "improve" God's food supply and get rid of the bitter taste in the fruit. By developing fruit that is sweeter and less bitter, we have damaged our food supply in two ways. We have reduced the B-17 (bitter) and have increased the sugar (sweet). This brings on a host of other diseases in addition to cancer. The Word of God reminds us that things sweet in the mouth may be bitter in the belly (Rev. 10:10). And of course things bitter in the mouth may be sweet in the belly! No doubt this Biblical truth has a physical warning for us as well as the spiritual message.

Of course, strong opposition has developed against vitamin B-17, but this is to be expected. As shown in an earlier chapter, man has always had organized opposition to all of God's natural health treatments. This is not likely to change, because the Word of God warns us that "evil men and seducers shall wax worse and worse" (2 Tim. 3:13). The opposition to Kreb's discovery has been especially strong because he, like Louis Pasteur before him, is a chemist and not a physician. Apparently both men encountered opposition for intruding into territory that others felt was their own.

EVIDENCE IN FAVOR OF VITAMIN B-17

I am often asked this question, "Do you really believe vitamin B-17 works?" Everybody seems to be looking for an *opinion* on every important question. So few people are willing to think for themselves, to examine evidence, and to arrive at logical conclusions. I try not to be an opinionated person myself, and I certainly do not want others to merely accept my conclusions without investigation. Often a person who hears of B-17 asks his doctor's opinion, gets a negative reply, and considers the matter settled. For the Christian, this is a disgrace and a sin. We are warned not to make decisions without investigating the facts (Prov. 18:13). We are warned to make righteous judgments. The Christian is responsible for investigating the facts, for asking God for wisdom to think straight, and for deciding wisely on the basis of the evidence. If we are too lazy to investigate and too lazy to think, then we will be tempted to ask the opinion of some so-called professional instead. But if we thus arrive at the wrong opinion, it may cost us our own life or the life of a loved one, and God will not hold us guiltless. Ignorance is no excuse when we have the opportunity to know the facts.

The evidence in favor of vitamin B-17 is similar to the evidence in favor of the trophoblast theory, for the two are closely related. I will give here the considerations that have led me to the firm conviction that B-17 is an effective natural anti-cancer agent.

The Testimony of Theology. The belief in an anti-cancer vitamin is consistent with the Word of God and our belief in a wise and good Creator. Since we know that God put vitamins in our environment to prevent many other chronic diseases, why not a vitamin against cancer also?

The Testimony of Biology. The body has natural methods of controlling the number of red blood cells so that normally we do not have too few or too many. The same is true of white blood cells. Is it not logical then that there are natural means of preventing an excess of malignant cells?

The Testimony of History. Every time in history that a natural means of combating disease has been developed, professional healers have used powerful methods to oppose it. In every important case it has turned out that the natural health advocates were right and the "orthodox" professionals were wrong. History always repeats itself. We have every reason to be confident that the final results will be the same in this case. As mentioned before, the Christian will have to believe that the ultimate opposition to God's methods of healing comes from Satan. This is part of the lesson of history.

The Testimony of Cytology. By the use of the microscope, researchers have been able to see cancer cells die when they come in contact with

B-17. Dr. Dean Burk was head of the cytochemistry section of the National Cancer Institute for many years. It has been reported that when he added B-17 to a cancer culture, he could see the cancer cells dying off like flies. Not one of them was able to survive. A look at his record would likely convince any unbiased person that Dr. Burk is America's top expert in the field of cytology (cell studies). But Dr. Burk's superiors were apparently career politicians, not scientists, and they did little or nothing about his discoveries.

The Testimony of Medical Anthropology. One important aspect of medical research is comparing the diseases in various parts of the world. This can reveal how our environment contributes to disease. And all over the world we find that where people eat a diet rich in B-17, they do not have cancer. The worlds' richest B-17 diet is found in Hunza. The principle crop in Hunza is the apricot and the most prized food is the apricot seed. The Hunzas eat 200 times as much B-17 as Americans do. Not one case of cancer has ever been found in Hunza. But when the natives leave Hunza and adopt a Western diet, then some of them have developed cancer. A similar pattern is found among the Eskimos of the far North and several African and Indian tribes. In every case these cancer-free peoples are known to have a diet rich in B-17.

The Testimony of Foreign Governments. Frequently I encounter a person who knows that

B-17 has not yet been approved by the U.S. Government. He then hastily concludes that it could not possibly be any good. How ignorant can you get? Is the American government the only government in the world? Do not other nations have just as much intelligence and just as much good sense as we do? Twenty-four major foreign governments have become convinced that B-17 is a useful anti-cancer substance and have approved its use. Are we stupid enough to believe that all these other governments are wrong and ours alone is right?

The Testimony of Famous Cancer Scientists. The enemies of B-17 often state that only quacks use this substance. Of course, they also said that vitamin C for scurvy was quackery from its discovery in 1535 until its adoption in 1795. But the truth is that several of the world's most renowned cancer scientists believe vitamin B-17 to be an effective anti-cancer agent. Included are such famous names as: Manuel D. Navarro, M.D., Manila; Ernesto Contreras, M.D., Tijuana, Mexico; Hans A. Nieper, M.D., Hanover, Germany; John A. Morrone, M.D., Jersey City, New Jersey; Dr. N. R. Bouziane, Montreal, Canada.

The Testimony of Common Experience. There are growing thousands of persons all over the world who have come to understand B-17 and to firmly believe in it. Many of them have now been on a B-17 rich diet for many years. So far there is no case on record of these persons contracting cancer. Even though God planned B-17 as a preventive and not a cure, thousands have had to turn to it for therapy nevertheless. Not every cancer patient is fortunate enough to find a physician who understands B-17. Many have to do the best they can and secure B-17 anywhere they can for their own metabolic needs. Many hundreds, perhaps thousands, have reported good results. Some have achieved remarkable results. I personally have known about 40 persons who used B-17. The great majority reported definite objective improvement. A few are alive and working long after they were supposed to be dead. A few seemed to receive little help. But of course we must keep in mind that most of these patients were far advanced, many were terminal and had been given up by orthodox practitioners. When you consider this fact, the results are most encouraging. Those who began taking B-17 earliest always got the best results.

The Testimony of Surgical Experience. Surgery is sometimes necessary for the cancer patient because the tumor is blocking a vital passage or is otherwise damaging a vital organ. It may be too late to attempt to dissolve the tumor. But many cancer surgeons still believe in B-17 and use it in conjunction with the surgery. They believe that B-17 treatments for a few weeks prior to surgery discourage the rapid spread of cancer that often follows cancer surgery. Now if B-17 minimizes the danger of post-operative cancer spread, why does it do so? Is this not further evidence the B-17 destroys malignant cells?

    I believe B-17 works. I have risked my life on this conviction. Of course I do not know to what extent it works, what the unknown variables may be, and what exceptions may exist. There is much yet to be learned. But B-17 is obviously an important part of God's anti-cancer mechanism. I thank God I learned about this and am able to encourage others with this conviction. If it took cancer to make me learn this, then I thank God for my cancer!

"In every thing give thanks"
(1 Thessalonians 5:18)

I can thank God for cancer, because it led me to understand this basic fact of human nature—

PRINCIPLE NO. 8: THE MAJORITY OPINION IS OFTEN ATHEISTIC AND WRONG

An acquaintance of mine once learned of my convictions on the natural control of cancer and exclaimed, "How can you believe that? Surely you don't know more than all those doctors!" Well, it isn't quite like that. This controversy does not put me alone on one side and all the physicians in the world on the other side. I realize that probably the majority of physicians in this country are on the other side of the fence, along with quite a few scientists, many politicians, and a lot of wealthy drug manufacturers. But I also realize that I am on the same side of the fence with a rapidly growing minority of American physicians, many physicians in other lands, and some of the world's most eminent scientists. I am also joined by a great host of Bible-believing Christians who believe that B-17 is of God and that the opposition to B-17 is not of God. So I am not alone by any means. Scores of others have written about B-17 long before I learned of it.

I am not the least bit afraid of being on the minority side of a controversy. History records that the majority has usually been wrong in every major controversy. Truth is always discovered by the minority and it is normal for the majority to resist because new truth disturbs its established behavior patterns. We can expect the majority to continue to be wrong as long as the majority continues to leave God out of its reasoning processes.

THE MEANING OF ATHEISM

It can be demonstrated that the majority opinion concerning B-17 is atheistic at its foundation. So first we must be sure that we understand the word *atheist*. The word is formed from two Greek words, *a* and *theos*. *Theos* refers to God as a person. The *a* is the common Greek negative prefix. It reverses the meaning of any word. This prefix can convey the ideas of absence, removal, opposition, and several other related negative concepts. So by its structure, the word *atheist* can mean denial of God's existence, the ignoring of God, effort to get rid of God, or opposition to God. Now one may feel that the common usage of the word refers to one who does not believe in the existence of God. But this cannot be the correct meaning of the term, for there are no such persons in the world! Does that shock you? Well, I mean just exactly that! God tells us in no uncertain terms that He has revealed Himself to all men in nature and that all men have seen the evidence of His existence (Rom. 1:18-20). I don't care how loudly a man claims to disbelieve in the existence of God. That man is not speaking his convictions, he is speaking his wishes! He is trying to get rid of the idea of God. But God says that the man is aware of His existence and I believe God. So the word *atheist* cannot refer to one who does not believe in God; it must have some other meaning.

God Himself gives us an understanding of what atheism really is. "The fool has said in his heart, [there is] no God" (Ps. 14:1). Notice that this fool did not say with his mouth that there was no God. He merely said in the Hebrew language "no God," and he said it in his heart.

That means that God was not taken into consideration in his reasoning or his emotions. God was not openly denied, He was just left out. That is the true nature of atheism. A man can be atheistic in one area of his life and not in another. Even a genuine Christian can be atheistic in some part of his life. For example a Christian might really have great faith in God to guide certain areas of his life, but he might neglect to bring God into his business life. So his business is atheistic, God is left out. Another might fail to consider God in his marriage. So his marriage is atheistic, God is left out. I feel certain that I know some physicians who are great Christians: they love God, they teach Bible classes and teach them well. But they leave God out of their medical reasonings. Their medical beliefs are dictated by "headquarters," and God is left out of this part of their life. So their medical practice is atheistic. The so-called scientific world has often made assumptions that were atheistic and which later turned out to be false. The saddest part of this is that God's children often accept these atheistic assumptions of science and go along with them blindly.

EXAMPLES OF ATHEISTIC ASSUMPTIONS OF SCIENCE

We live in a society that almost worships science. Like most other Americans, I have always felt a sense of awe at the remarkable accomplishments of the scientific world. This reverence needs to be tempered with an understanding of the weaknesses and limitations of science. We need to realize that what is called science is often not science at all. The word *science* is from the Latin *scio* meaning *to know*. Therefore *science* actually means *knowledge*. But so-called science is constantly changing. That which is taught as science in one generation is discovered to be false in the next generation. This has always been the case. If it is proved to be false, then it was not knowledge and was therefore not science. It is vitally important to realize that much of what is called science today will be proved false tomorrow. So science is not God, as many people seem to think.

Why is it that science has been so full of error and continues to be so? One reason is that all reasoning, including scientific reasoning, must begin somewhere. There must be some basic assumptions. If these basic assumptions are incorrect, then the experimentation, research, and the conclusions that follow can all be fruitless. And when God is left out of these basic assumptions, they are likely to be incorrect. No amount of laboratory measurement can compensate for this original error.

For example, astronomy was considered a well-developed science 500 years ago. However, the greatest astronomers just assumed that the earth was flat, that it was held up by some structural support, and that it was the center of the universe. All these assumptions were false and led to enormous confusion. Why did the scientists make these false assumptions? Because they left God out of their assumptions. If they had carefully read the Word of God, they would not have made any of these errors. Many astronomers of that day had a vast intellect, some were mathematical wizards, and they developed instruments to measure the position and movements of the planets. From this they were able to determine the exact time of an eclipse hundreds of years in advance. So they were extremely skillful. Still they blundered terribly and damaged the very science that they loved. Why? They left God out of their basic assumptions.

The tragedy of such error is enormous. Once an error like this is established, it becomes institutionalized. Vested interests develop around it and there is powerful resistance to any change. Those who discover the truth and challenge the error are branded as heretics and troublemakers worthy of severe punishment. For example, the great Italian philosopher Giordano Bruno was burned at the stake in 1600 for teaching that the world was round. Galileo was imprisoned for similar teachings, as were many others. Even though the murderers of Bruno were the religious authorities of Rome, they were supporting a false view of science that was atheistic at its foundation. You see, religious people are often atheistic too! We must realize that once a "scientific" error is accepted and institutionalized, it can only be uprooted with extreme difficulty. The mere discovery of the truth does not remove the error, for those who have built a career on the error will defend that career with all their might. The Bible teaches us that men are not so much interested in discovering truth as they are in protecting their own jobs, their own reputation, and their own power.

Many people have the idea that even if researchers make a false assumption, later laboratory research will correct this. Many times this does not happen. For example, the theory of evolution is a classic case of incorrectable error. Charles Darwin proposed the theory, admitted it was just a theory, and offered no proof that man evolved from lower forms of life. This was an atheistic assumption. The so-called scientific world eagerly accepted this false assumption without proof. Why? Man is a sinner and would like to get rid of God. Since that time we have had tens of thousands of "scientists" spending billions of dollars in thousands of laboratories trying to discover the details of *how* man evolved. Now just think, how long will it take them to discover how man evolved? Of course they will never get the answer in ten million years of research because *man did not evolve, he was created!* You see, once a false atheistic assumption is accepted, all future research based on this assumption is useless and may never correct the original error.

This should help us to realize that we must abandon our reverence for "scientific research." No matter how many men we put on a research project, no matter how much money we spend, no matter how sophisticated the equipment, can all be to no avail if the basic assumptions are incorrect. And they will be incorrect if they are atheistic, if God is left out. The Lord warns us of this endless, fruitless search for truth in 2 Tim. 3:7. Men shall be "ever learning, but never able to come to the knowledge of the truth." Also we must realize that what is called *science* is often not science at all. Research in the field of "evolution" is not science no matter what men call it, for science is truth and knowledge. Since the basic assumptions of evolution are not true, the resulting research cannot correctly be called *knowledge* or *science*. The Bible warns us of those who work against God, using "oppositions of science falsely so called" (1 Tim. 6:20). Plainly then there is much propaganda today that claims to be science but is not science at all and is definitely against God.

THE DISGRACEFUL FAILURE OF ORTHODOX CANCER TREATMENTS

Whatever one may believe about natural cancer treatments, one thing is quite clear. No one was ever killed by using natural foods.

Orthodox medicine certainly would not make such a claim for the deadly methods they use. There is a rapidly growing realization among the public and also among the physicians that presently recognized cancer therapies are generally a failure. We are hearing of more and more physicians and nurses who will admit this to their trusted friends. We frequently hear medical circles boast of a long-term survival record of 30%. Such figures are misleading to say the least, for most of these are skin cancer patients. Apparently radiation has been of some help to some skin cancer patients. But what about the serious problem of internal metastasized cancer? The records indicate that only about *one in a thousand* of these is being saved by currently approved methods.

There is another tragedy that clearly points out the failure and the disgraceful conduct of the modern cancer industry. I refer to the current scandal surrounding the breast cancer controversy. For several decades now, multitudes of women have been railroaded into a complete mastectomy without being warned of the serious consequences and without being told of the possible alternatives. The surgeon made the decision and did not allow the patient to have the needed information or to participate in the decision. This matter has become so serious that some states have enacted legislation compelling the physician to reveal both dangers and alternatives so that the patient can make a wiser decision. If it is now a crime to withhold this vital information from the patient, then it always was a crime in the sight of God! Can you imagine the law having to compel surgeons to give information to patients? Obviously the lawmakers in these states believe that past secrecy has been cruel to the patients. From the Biblical point of view we must realize that to withhold important information is deception, and deception is lying. Therefore it is obvious that hundreds of thousands of women have been lied to concerning breast surgery! They have been led to believe that they had no alternative to a complete mastectomy. They have also been led to believe that there would be no serious consequences from such a procedure. There are now thousands of these mutilated women who are awakening to the sad reality. Many of them are now bitter because they feel that the mutilation was cruel and did not help the situation. A growing number of surgeons now claim that the removal of the breast does no more good than the removal of the lump. This writer heard one prominent California physician, speaking before a large audience, proclaim with firm conviction that he had observed for years that breast cancer patients who had no treatment at all survived longer than those who had surgery, radiation, and chemotherapy! If the patients did just as well on *no treatment,* we wonder what great results might have been accomplished if they had been on thorough orthodox treatment and then die. A nurse recently called my home to tell of her own personal experience. Four years ago she discovered that she had cancer of the breast, and she decided to do nothing about it. When asked why, she explained that she had seen several members of her family go through the endless agony of cutting, burning, and poisoning. She said she would rather die naturally than go through what her loved ones had gone through. She also stated that in the four years since her diagnosis, her condition had gotten no worse. This is not an isolated case. We are encountering this same attitude more and more frequently. These statements are not designed to give advice concerning any individual case, for individual cases differ. These statements do not imply that no one is ever helped by orthodox methods. But these facts illustrate that the public is becoming more and more aware of the poor record of orthodox treatments. The fact that such books can be written and that such statements are frequently made is itself evidence of the failure of the cancer industry. And why this tragic failure? The most obvious cause of the failure is the fact that the whole system is based on the atheistic assumption that God has no regular anti-cancer system.

In this connection it is important for the reader to understand the basis of medical practice. Medical practice is not based entirely on medical science, as many suppose. Current metabolic therapy (controlling the body chemistry by the use of natural substances).

A competent medical researcher is now in the process of writing a book comparing the survival of treated and non-treated cancer patients. He is going to try to prove by statistics that non-treated cancer patients are now surviving much longer on the average than those patients who follow the standard route of surgery, radiation, and chemotherapy to the cemetery. I have not seen his statistics and am certainly not competent to express an opinion on his thesis. But it will be most interesting to study his work when it is published. This much we do know, that a growing number of common people are coming to the same conclusion after watching several of their loved ones go through medical practice is based partly on medical art, partly on medical science, but mostly on medical philosophy, medical economics, and medical politics. When the medical philosophy is atheistic, the medical science can be futile, and the medical practice can be worthless or even harmful. For this reason there has been a long-standing saying among the other sciences that "medical science is the most unscientific of all sciences." History has confirmed the truth of this statement.

This is not to imply that all medical men are guilty of these errors. By no means! There are a growing number of practitioners who realize the sad history of their profession and who earnestly desire to break out of this pattern. Apparently they are still in the minority, and it is not easy for them to overcome the powerful pressure to conform that is put on them by the organization. This is according to our thesis. The majority is usually wrong, but thank God for that minority who is trying to hold out for the truth!

Why do these errors persist? It is because the atheistic majority is organized and powerful. They resist change for economic reasons. Vested interests are at stake. History has confirmed this sad fact again and again.

A most shocking fact comes to light when we compare the currently popular cancer therapies with the practices of pagan witch doctors for centuries past. When a devil-worshipping witch doctor had a really serious case, how did he treat the patient? Historically, the most powerful medicines of the witch doctor, reserved for the difficult cases, have been cutting with knives, burning with fire, and poisoning with toxic substances. These severe methods have supposedly been capable of driving out the most difficult disease, that is, if they did not kill the patient first. You say, "How ignorant! How disgusting!" Right, but how is cancer treated today in "enlightened" America? By cutting, burning, and poisoning! These severe methods are supposedly capable of controlling cancer, that is, if they do not kill the patient first!

I can hear someone exclaim, "But this comparison is not fair!" Some will feel that even though the treatments are similar, that there is a difference in the results. We may feel that current cancer treatments do have *some success* and that the witch doctor had *no success*. But what proof do we have of this? Multitudes of the witch doctor's followers were absolutely certain that he got good results in some cases. Can we prove he did not? Of course not! I am not insisting that the results are exactly the same in both cases. But I do contend that we do not know for sure how much better one is than the other. The important point is that the two treatments are so *similar*. Why? Could it be because the majority atheistic opinion has a tendency to revert to ancient paganism?

THE ATHEISTIC FOUNDATION OF THE MODERN CANCER INDUSTRY

No doubt all of my readers will now admit that so-called science, including medical science, has blundered terribly in the past because of false atheistic assumptions. But many of us are tempted to think that this could not happen today. On what basis can we conclude that modern man is free from the godless errors of the past? The Word of God does not teach that man will stop his godless reasonings. On the contrary, we are plainly told that "evil men and seducers shall wax worse and worse." We are warned that in the last days men shall have a form of godliness, but shall deny the power of God (2 Tim. 3:5). In other words, even religious persons shall deny the powerful things that God is doing. So any Bible-believing Christian should realize that the atheistic assumptions of science are still taking place, with disastrous results.

Let us take a look at the modern cancer industry, a very lucrative 12 billion dollars a year industry. A little investigation and thought will reveal that this industry is not based so much on science, but on an atheistic assumption. At its very foundation, the cancer business today assumes that God did not plan any cancer-fighting mechanisms in nature. That is an atheistic assumption. If this assumption is an error, as millions are firmly convinced that it is, then think of the enormous consequences! The cancer industry will make no effort to discover the cancer-fighting substances in our natural environment, and will seek to fight cancer only with man-made methods! It is clearly apparent that such a godless assumption has been made because for many years the cancer industry has parroted this motto, "No food and no combination of foods can alter the course of cancer." Notice the profound significance of this assumption! This means that God did not put any natural anti-cancer materials in our environment. This atheistic assumption has led to the conclusion that cancer can be treated only with surgery, radiation, or chemotherapy (cutting, burning, or poisoning).

There is another tragic situation that proves

clearly that such an atheistic assumption has been made. All over America the established cancer business has tried to make it illegal to treat cancer by the use of natural substances. Several states, several government agencies, and almost all organized medicine in this country has gone with this persecution. The mere existence of such opposition is clear evidence that our cancer industry is assuming, without proof, that there are no anti-cancer materials in nature. This is an atheistic assumption.

Look at the monstrous evil that can result from such an atheistic assumption. Since the authorities have ruled that no natural anti-cancer substances exist, it therefore becomes illegal to even look for them! So God is ruled out before the search even begins.

Now let us consider the alternative. Suppose our "cancer authorities" had assumed at the beginning that God may have put some cancer-fighting materials in our environment. Then they would have looked earnestly for such materials and would have encouraged others to do the same. Those who made any progress in the search would have been rewarded. This search would have led to simpler, more natural, less expensive cancer treatments that cooperated with nature instead of working against nature. The only disadvantage of this approach, if it can be considered a disadvantage, is that it is less profitable as a business. It is more

God-honoring and, we are convinced, more effective.

This should be sufficient to convince the reader that modern medical practice is not necessarily based on science. The so-called science must be based on some assumption. The original assumption determines the course of the "scientific research" and the nature of the medical practice. Since America's cancer industry is founded on atheism, the true Christian can not have much confidence in it.

For many of us it has been a disturbing experience to learn that the majority is usually wrong. And why are they wrong? They leave God out of their reasonings. As the Scripture says, "God is not in all his thoughts" (Ps. 10:4). What shall we do then? Are we going to continue to follow the crowd? Are we going to try to "get on the band wagon"? Are we going to continue to assume that the crowd is right because they are in the majority? As for me, I have learned better. I will believe that God has anti-cancer mechanisms in nature, even if I am in the minority. I thank God that I have learned this lesson!

"In every thing give thanks"
(1 Thessalonians 5:18)

I can thank God for cancer, for it awakened me to this frightening political principle—

PRINCIPLE NO. 9: IT IS "ILLEGAL" FOR GOD TO RELIEVE CANCER MISERY

Do you find the title of this principle sickening and horrible? Well, it is true in a very real sense, but it does need some clarification. Practically every natural cancer treatment ever discovered in America has been made illegal to some extent, and remember that *natural* means *God-given*. So when natural methods are outlawed, then God's methods are outlawed.

There are powerful elements in our medical-industrial-drug establishment that are determined to protect their lucrative cancer monopoly at all costs. And since God's methods of natural treatment remain an ever-present threat to their vast revenues, then such treatments must be stopped. Their favorite method is to use the law as a tool to protect their monopoly. These attempts to make natural cancer treatments illegal have not been 100 percent successful, but even where natural treatments are not illegal, the opposition falsely claims they are illegal in order to discourage their use.

So we are completely justified in using this title for this chapter because the avowed goal of the enemy is the complete illegality of all God-given cancer treatments, and the goal has been largely reached.

THE BACKGROUND OF THE LEGAL PROBLEMS

One may well wonder how such a monstrous evil could ever come to pass. How could lawmakers and the general public ever be persuaded to accept such wicked legislation? The answer is simple. It all began with the atheistic assumption discussed in the preceding chapter. Decades ago, when certain medical researchers began to develop natural treatments for cancer, many orthodox physicians just assumed that there were no natural anti-cancer materials in our environment. On the basis of such an assumption, it logically followed that the promoters of such treatments were quacks. Government agencies accepted this falsehood, and laws and regulations against such treatments soon followed. But please notice that all this logic began with an atheistic assumption. No doubt some of these militant "anti-quack" persons were well-meaning. But as we have seen, a well-meaning person who reasons without God can set in motion a tragic chain of events. The people who crucified Jesus no doubt thought in their own twisted minds that they were right. But this does not reduce their guilt. They could have known the truth, had they been willing to know the truth. And the men who crucified the God-given cancer treatments are not guiltless just because some of them may have thought they were doing right. They should not have assumed that God could not create a cancer control. No matter how sincere their intentions, they are guilty of the high crime of atheistic assumption which results in rebellion against the plan of the Creator. It has often been said that "the road to Hell is paved with good intentions." This may be a very accurate description of any "good intentions" that started the legal opposition to natural cancer therapy.

If some of the early suspicion of natural remedies was sincere, the vicious opposition that soon developed was quite otherwise. The monstrous evil of harassment, threats, and dishonest legal shenanigans against natural or non-toxic therapies that developed is the saddest chapter in American history. This gruesome story is told in detail and is thoroughly documented by Suzanne Caum in *Cancer Cures Crucified*. We will only review the sad story briefly here.

In 1917, Dr. William Koch was a highly competent physician and biochemist in Detroit, Michigan. He was instructor of Histology and Embryology at the University of Michigan. He was also professor of Physiology at Wayne State University and Pathologist in Detroit Women's Hospital. With these eminent qualifications he was highly regarded by his colleagues until he developed a successful cancer treatment using glyoxylide. Then all of a sudden he became a "quack" and an imposter in the opinion of his medical society. The fact that he was saving lives that had been given up by other physicians made no difference. He was considered a serious economic threat and they were out to get him at all costs. After a prolonged period of lies, false charges, false witnesses, and unconstitutional maneuvers, he was finally put out of business in America. He then went to Brazil where thousands of cancer patients in this country were sacrificed in order to protect the pride and economic security of his colleagues.

From 1946 to 1959, Dr. Max Gerson of New

York City successfully treated many cancer patients using a strict nutritional approach. Hundreds of patients testified and told of the benefits they received from the Gerson treatment after orthodox methods had failed. He was sent to jail and died soon after his release.

Dr. Andrew Ivy of Chicago developed a non-toxic treatment around 1951 which he called Krebiozin. Over 10,000 patients benefited from his treatment. The government refused to issue him a $50,000 grant to develop his treatment, but they later spent over $1,000,000 on a trial trying to send him to prison. The presiding judge caught government witnesses telling falsehoods in the trial. Dr. Ivy was acquitted. The Illinois medical authorities nevertheless have continued their efforts to destroy him.

Dr. Harry Hoxsey of Dallas, Texas, developed a highly successful cancer treatment using a combination of herbs and other substances. Beginning about 1936, he treated over 10,000 patients, and a large percentage of these patients claimed to be cured or helped. The medical establishment carried him to court twenty times in an effort to stop his practice, but he won all twenty cases. This type of persecution never stops. They finally got Dr. Hoxsey. How? At his twenty-first lawsuit many persons testified of the benefits they had received from his treatment. However the court ruled that these persons were not medical experts and therefore their opinions were of no value. So their testimony was not admitted as evidence. Because the court admitted the evidence against him (given by his enemies of course) and would not admit the abundant evidence for him, naturally he lost the case. Is this constitutional? Is such legal maneuvering consistent with the principle of fairness and freedom on which this country was built? Dr. Hoxsey, driven out of practice in this country, moved to Mexico where he continued to help cancer patients with his God-given method for many years.

This list goes on and on almost indefinitely. There are at least twenty physicians in the history of this country who have developed similar natural cancer therapies. All have been persecuted by medical societies and government agencies. In no case has their treatment been tested by the authorities. In every case they have been charged with "quackery." They have been assumed guilty and they have been persecuted without any effort being made to discover the truth about their treatment. But let us come to what is probably the last and greatest episode in this ugly fight against God-given cancer remedies.

During the 1950's, Dr. Ernst T. Krebs, Jr., a San Francisco biochemist, proved that vitamin B-17, a natural substance found in over 1,000 growing plants, would destroy cancer cells but was harmless to non-cancerous cells. Many top scientists in other parts of the world confirmed

Krebs' theory. It is important for the reader to understand that the vitamin B-17 treatment is totally different from the many other non-toxic treatments we have mentioned. These other treatments undoubtedly have some value because so many patients testified of the benefits received. But the exact biological or chemical method by which they fought cancer was not known or at least not revealed to the public. Not so with vitamin B-17. Top biochemists in many countries are in perfect agreement as to exactly how amygdalin works. As previously discussed, the enzymes in the malignant cell are different from the enzymes in a non-cancerous cell. Because of this, B-17 releases cyanide in cancer cells but is harmless to and actually nourishes ordinary cells. This is such a wonderful design of nature that it just had to be planned by a good and wise Creator.

During the early years of B-17 use against cancer, there were some very successful cases, even though there was much to be learned about the size of dosage, method of administration, and the like. Usually no one would try B-17 until all other methods had failed and death was near. Even so, there were a number of patients who improved remarkably on the treatment. Much of this early B-17 experience was in the state of Califronia where its value against cancer was first discovered. As soon as these successful treatments began to be publicized, the California medical authorities set in motion their machinery to stop this new threat to their cancer monopoly. The Cancer Commission of the California Medical Association, consisting of some nine doctors, was appointed to "investigate" the Laetrile treatment. Of course these men were cancer "specialists," and cancer specialists usually earn huge incomes from orthodox cancer treatments. In any other situation, it would be understood that such men were not in position to render an impartial verdict. To make matters worse, this committee turned the investigation over to the committee chairman and secretary, Dr. McDonald and Dr. Garland. These two men never used B-17, but based their report on the records of other researchers. They concluded that Laetrile was of no value in the treatment of cancer. Their report was never signed, but the full committee accepted it, and the California Medical Association accepted it. On the basis of this spurious report, the California legislature enacted a law forbidding the use of vitamin B-17 in "arresting, curing, or alleviating cancer."

As cruel and unreasonable and unconstitutional as this law was, it was limited in its scope. It applied only to physicians, and only then when the vitamin was used as a specific for cancer. Notice that the law did not forbid the use of B-17 in the treatment of other diseases and in the improvement of general health, as it had been used for centuries. Notice also that the law did not forbid the manufacture, sale, or use of

B-17 by ordinary citizens. And most of all, notice that this law covered only one state, California.

The application of a foolish law can often be infinitely more foolish than the law itself. Such was certainly the case in this situation. On the basis of this California law, the U.S. Food and Drug Administration began a campaign of harassment to prevent the use of vitamin B-17 *for any purpose in any state!* Notice the cruelty and absurdity of it all! This is an example of how the opposition to natural cancer treatments becomes more and more unreasonable and unfair as more and more agencies get involved in the fight.

In order for the reader to understand the shallow foundation of this FDA opposition, we will summarize here the fallacies in the development of the opposition.

1) The two doctors who wrote the California report had no personal knowledge of vitamin B-17 (Laetrile).

2) It was later proved that they had falsified the records of the researchers.

3) They did not sign the report. Was this a device to slander B-17 and yet escape prosecution if their falsehoods were discovered?

4) Dr. McDonald, the committee chairman, is the same man who testified before the Surgeon-General that cigarette smoking would prevent lung cancer. This demonstrates the

degree of scientific ability possessed by the investigators.

5) Most of the patients in the test were near death at the time B-17 was administered. The amount given was about two grams each. It usually takes about 100 grams to bring cancer under control.

6) The full membership of the Cancer Commission accepted this flimsy unsigned report without investigation.

7) The California Medical Association accepted the recommendation of the commission without investigation.

8) The California Legislature accepted the urging of the medical "authorities" and enacted anti-Laetrile legislation without any investigation.

9) The U.S. Food and Drug Administration has attempted to force this state law on the entire nation. There is no Federal law against B-17.

10) The FDA has tried to ban the use of B-17 for all purposes, even though the California law only mentions cancer.

11) The FDA has tried to prevent all citizens from purchasing or using B-17 even though the California law only refers to physicians.

So much for the absurdities! The reader should realize by now what we are up against when we try to use God's remedies for cancer. The FDA and other government agencies wage war on these natural substances, *not because the law requires it, but because they want to.* Any flimsy law is used as an excuse for the action, then is applied completely out of proportion to the original intent of the lawmaker.

The reader can easily see the cruelty and folly of this harassment by making a comparison. Some cancer patients take aspirin to relieve cancer pain, just as many also use B-17 to relieve cancer pain. Now suppose some state passes a law forbidding doctors to use aspirin in the relief of cancer. That would be an absolutely ridiculous law. But then suppose the FDA, on the basis of that law, forbids anyone, anywhere, in any state to use aspirin for any purpose whatever! Suppose they seized all existing stocks of aspirin and arrested any doctor who used it? You say, "Such a thing could not happen!" Oh, yes, it can and it has happened! That's exactly what happened to vitamin B-17, and I will defy anyone to give any reasonable explanation why B-17 does not deserve as much freedom as aspirin! In fact, B-17 should have more freedom than aspirin because aspirin kills at least 100 persons annually in this country and there is no case on record of B-17 ever hurting anyone! Any person who would be opposed to forbidding aspirin but in favor of forbidding B-17 must be ignorant or else a hypocrite! I don't see how we could possibly arrive at any other conclusion!

I can hear someone reply, "But I really don't believe B-17 has any value against cancer. I'm sincere. I think B-17 should be banned because I feel it has no value." That makes no difference! Such a person is still a hypocrite, because there are thousands of useless drugs on the market and he doesn't try to ban them! There are many physicians who believe that aspirin is worthless, but it is not forbidden! We are dishonest when we apply a system of logic to one situation and do not apply it to another situation. Any honest person would be in favor of making B-17 legal even if it had no value whatever. That would give it equal standing with other reportedly useless preparations. But vitamin B-17 does have value, much value, as dozens of top scientists the world over have proved and thousands of patients have learned by experience!

From these historical facts it is obvious that there is a determined effort on the part of powerful forces in our medical establishment to prevent the use of any natural cancer treatment. It makes no difference that their own methods fail, these are the only methods that can be permitted. It matters not that the natural treatments are successful, they must be stopped at all costs. Only three basic treatments are allowed: surgery, radiation, and chemotherapy. All three of these are miserable failures, as thousands of physicians will admit. In addition, all three of these methods are highly destructive to the body, again as thousands of physicians will admit.

We may wonder what is the criterion by which the medical establishment measures a cancer therapy. How do they decide which new therapies they will accept? The facts give a clean answer. It is crystal clear that effectiveness is not a criterion, for the effective treatments have generally been banned and the harmful treatments have generally been accepted. The answer is clear. In order for a cancer treatment to be accepted by the medical establishment, *it must be harmful to the human body!* Poisonous chemicals by the dozen have been approved for use in chemotherapy. But if a substance is natural and non-poisonous, it is doomed from the beginning no matter how much evidence there is to support it!

Can a cancer cure be found and put into general use in this country? Absolutely not! Not under the present circumstances. None of the accepted therapies are very successful. The true control of cancer is obviously in natural methods, but these are all illegal. We are then driven to this inescapable conclusion:

IT IS A CRIME IN AMERICA TO DISCOVER A CURE FOR CANCER!

Since any successful cancer treatment is obviously going to be natural and non-toxic, and since such treatments are illegal, then God has been ruled out of the cancer business in America. We may well wonder if the wrath of Almighty God against his great national evil is not already falling on our land! We may cry out about the 1000 cancer patients who die nedlessly every day in this country. But don't blame God! He put the preventive in nature. Blame the politicians and the cancer monopoly that wants to protect its 12 billion dollars annual income!

OPPOSITION CLAIMS EXAMINED

We are now ready to examine the excuses that are sometimes given by the opposition to justify their war against vitamin B-17. But first it would be good to identify the opposition. Most resistance to B-17 and other natural cancer remedies comes from the American Medical Association and their state and county affiliates, the Food and Drug Administration, and the American Cancer Society. Sometimes other government agencies are enlisted in the campaign of harassment. There is abundant evidence to indicate that a vast international drug and chemical cartel is the real power behind the opposition. If the reader is interested in seeing documented proof of this, it is available in the reading list given at the close of this book.

When these enemies of natural healing seek to make B-17 illegal, what excuses do they give for such action? Their argument consists of several accusations, each of which will deceive the simple, but all of which are totally absurd when examined in the light of the facts. Here are the arguments:

They Claim That Physicians Who Use Laetrile Are Quacks. This is not a mistake, but an outright lie. The dictionary definition of a *quack* is one who professes to have knowledge which he does not have. The physicians who use B-17 are highly familiar with orthodox cancer treatments. In addition, they have gone further and have learned of nature's chemical wonders against malignancy. On the other hand, those who condemn B-17 are those who have not really investigated it. Who then are the real quacks? If I were a physician with the miserably poor record of cancer cures that most physicians have, I certainly would not call someone a quack who was having more success than I.

It is strange that these world famous physicians were eminently qualified and highly respected before they began to have success with B-17. Why is it that such success always turns a brilliant research scientist into a "quack"? The list of world-famous physicians who are currently having success with B-17 includes such names as:

HANS A. NIEPER, M.D., of Hanover, Germany, metabolism specialist and consultant to NASA. He has worked with the German Research Council, a government organization, and has published more than 200 papers. He played a major role in the development of cobalt therapy. He has used amygdalin since 1966 and says:

> Amygdalin appears to be very effective in the greater number of patients because it is non-toxic, can be used indefinitely, and does not conflict with other types of treatment such as radiation and surgery. There is an improvement of the general condition of the patients in almost all cases. The effect increases with the time for which it is given.

JOHN A. MORRONE, M.D., attending surgeon, Jersey City Medical Center, said in 1962:

> The use of Amygdalin intravenously in 10 cases of inoperable cancer, all with metastases, provided a dramatic relief from pain, control of fetor, and improved appetite.

N. R. BOUZIANE, M.D., Director, Research Laboratories, Saint Jeanne D'Arc Hospital in Montreal, former Professor of Clinical Pathology at the University of Montreal, and Dean of the American Society of Bio-Analysts, said that:

> In most cases, if not in all, pain diminishes and very often disappears. Patients under narcotics, morphine because there is no other therapy left for them, experience with amygdalin no further need for morphine, or at most a very small quantity.

MANUEL D. NAVARRO, M.D., Oncologist, Professor, Faculty of Medicine and Surgery,

University of Santo Tomas, Manila, Philippines. Having administered amygdalin to patients since 1954, many of them terminal, Dr. Navarro now says:

> Of all the therapeutic effects of amygdalin in cancer, the relief of pain is the first thing the patient notices. This is due to the analgesic actions of both the HCN and the benzaldehyde released at the cancer site. I have had several patients who needed morphine or Demerol to relieve pain. But they had better relief when amygdalin was given. The relief lasts from 18 to 24 hours or longer. What is more important, amygdalin is also anti-blastic. And because the pain is relieved, the patient develops an appetite and subsequently gains weight.

ERNESTO CONTERAS, M.D., Pathologist and Oncologist at the Clinica de Oncologia, Playas de Tijuana, Mexico, has administered amygdalin to thousands of cancer patients since 1964. He was Assistant Professor of Histology and Pathology in the Army Medical School, Mexico City, for 10 years until 1953 when he was appointed Chief Pathologist of the Army Military Hospital, Mexico City. He says:

> My experience in 10 years using amygdalin in terminal cancer patients is that in at least 60% of the cases it produces a striking analgesic effect and well-being sensation. I cannot say amygdalin is stronger than codeine and

morphine as a pain killer, but I can certainly state that in our clinic and hospital we very seldom use morphine or Demerol, and from the patients who come to us already addicted to these drugs, we are able to withdraw them in a short period of time.

I am personally acquainted with several physicians who have recently begun to use B-17 on cancer patients with good success. All of these men are honest, dedicated physicians. All are in good standing with their respective medical societies. All have previously used the standard approved methods of cancer therapy and are thoroughly familiar with the successes and failures of such methods. All are thrilled and delighted at the results they are now getting with B-17. None are promising miracles. None are advertising for patients. All are humble men who realize there is yet much to be learned about the most efficient use of B-17. But all are getting very encouraging results. It now remains to be seen if they will remain in good standing with their medical societies.

Now I ask the reader a question. Are these men to be branded as quacks just because they are using a new method? Don't forget that the first physicians to cure scurvy with vitamin C were called quacks also. I don't know about you, but I am quite sure who the real quacks are! We should also remember that the religious authorities who crucified Jesus used similar

charges against Him. In the language of that day He was branded a religious quack by those who were in power. But who were the real quacks?
They Claim That Vitamin B-17 May Be Toxic. This too is a deliberate falsehood, because the non-toxic character of B-17 has been known for centuries. The old name of this vitamin, *amygdalin*, is listed in standard pharmacology books as non-toxic as far back as 1840. It has long been used as a treatment for many diseases, including high blood pressure and allergies. Why did it suddenly gain the reputation of being toxic just at the time its cancer-fighting properties were discovered? The argument is often given that B-17 is toxic because the molecule contains the cyanide group. But every high school chemistry student knows better than this. Every molecule of common table salt contains one atom of deadly poisonous chlorine. But we are not afraid of table salt, because we know that the chlorine atom is locked in the molecule and is therefore harmless. Likewise both chemical theory and experience have proved that the cyanide group is safely locked in the B-17 molecule and is therefore harmless. But as previously explained, God has placed a special enzyme in the cancer cell that does release the cyanide group. So B-17 is toxic only to the cancer cells! Of course, toxicity is a relative matter. All substances are toxic to some degree if consumed in large enough quantities. This is true even of oxygen.

Common aspirin is 20 times more toxic than vitamin B-17. Even table sugar is toxic than B-17, as Dr. Dean Burk has clearly demonstrated.

In their absurd attempts to frighten the public away from B-17, the opposition has attempted to warn the public of the danger of eating apricot kernels, the richest natural source of the vitamin. Supplies of the seeds have been seized from the shelves of health food stores (unconstitutionally, of course). A popular television series, a propaganda tool of the medical establishment, presented a program in which a boy was found in a coma from eating peach kernels. Such nonsense! Such deception! I personally eat apricot or peach kernels every day, sometimes as many as 75 in one day. I have never experienced the slightest ill effects. In fact, the more I eat, the better I feel. Thousands of others have made the same discovery.

The most absurd part of this "toxic" accusation is this: the people who seek to make B-17 illegal on the grounds that it may be toxic are the same people who have approved dozens of deadly poisons for use in cancer chemotherapy. It would be hard to find anything in all of human history more hypocritical than this!

They Claim That Vitamin B-17 Should Not Be Approved Because It Has Not Been Sufficiently Tested. This is more hypocrisy for two reasons. First, the advocates of Laetrile have fought a frustrating battle for 23 years attempting to get the FDA to approve B-17 tests on human beings. The story of double-talk, trickery, and maneuvering that has blocked these tests is almost unbelievable. The agency that refuses to approve B-17 because it has not been sufficiently tested is the *same agency* that blocks such testing. For those who wish to read the full story of this fantastic conspiracy, see the reading list at the end of this book.

The second reason that such a claim is hypocritical is this: hundreds of other substances, many of them poisonous, have been approved for use in food and drugs without even being tested. Why is B-17 singled out for such close screening? The only possible answer to this question is that B-17 is a threat to the cancer monopoly. The charge of "not sufficiently tested" is a subterfuge. It *has been tested* by thousands of patients and hundreds of doctors in America and around the world!

They Claim That B-17 Therapy Should Not Be Approved Because This Might Cause Some Patients to Forego Approved Therapies. This is the most absurd and hypocritical of all the false charges. This is saying that a patient should not be allowed to use God's harmless remedies, because he might therefore fail to use man's expensive and destructive treatments! Why not? If a patient and his doctor choose to use natural treatments, why not let them? Whose business is it? Who would be harmed by such a freedom of choice? I cannot conceive of anyone opposing a man's freedom to choose his own therapy—unless, of course, his own economic welfare was threatened. I challenge anyone to give a reasonable explanation for denying a man and his doctor the right to use God-given food substances in any health treatment they desire. No one—and I do mean no one—will try to take this freedom away from the public except those who are making money from other therapies! There is no other explanation except the protection of a cancer industry monopoly. I am sorry this terrible thing is true in our land. But since it is true, I am glad that God allowed me to become aware of it. We need to see clearly the monstrous cruelty of those who want to force "approved" treatments on cancer patients and to deny them God-given natural treatments. Just remember that many orthodox physicians who are not friends of Laetrile have admitted that all currently approved methods of cancer treatment are failures! So the anti-Laetrile forces are trying to compel cancer patients to use treatments that are known to be practically useless!

I trust that by now the reader has seen the total lack of logic behind the anti-Laetrile arguments. It is impossible to believe that men in high positions can be that stupid. The only alternative is to believe that someone is promoting propaganda which they know to be false. The anti-Laetrile arguments are perfectly nil. In all human history there could not be an argument with such total lack of foundation!

They Claim That Laetrile Therapy Has Poor Records. The FDA says that they cannot approve B-17 until it is tested in "approved" hospitals by "approved" physicians. This, of course, means members of the AMA. But any such physician who dares to try B-17 is immediately ostracized and persecuted. How can we ever get good records under these circumstances? The people that demand good research and good records are the same people who prevented the research and the records in the first place.

They Claim That Laetrile Physicians Are Just Getting People's Money. This is too absurd a lie to deserve much discussion. The average cancer patient using "orthodox" treatments spends $15,000 or more and what does he get for it? A seven percent chance to live five years, according to American Cancer Society statistics. I personally have seen over twenty terminal cancer patients who have recovered by the use of B-17, and a few of these were close personal friends. Usually they spent only a few hundred dollars for the material. The busiest Laetrile physician I know has his patients order their own B-17 and he charges them only $1.00 for the injection. If a cancer patient gets on B-17 too late, he will very likely expire before he could spend $2,000 on B-17. If he gets on it early, he will very likely bring his cancer under control before he could spend $2,000. Now who is getting whose money?

They Claim That B-17 Gives False Hopes. Let us see who is guilty of giving false hopes. We have all seen many persons die of cancer soon after the cancer surgeon told them he "got it all." This statement is false and also is a form of deception to raise false hopes. No surgeon can get it all because removing a tumor does not cure the disease. It only removes a symptom. Experience has shown that in most cases the disease of cancer breaks out somewhere else after the removal of a tumor. Therefore when the surgeon tells the patient that he got it all, he is deceiving the patient into thinking the disease is cured when this is far from the truth. In many cases the cancer develops more rapidly after surgery. Is this not false hope of the worst kind? Any surgeon who misleads a patient with false hope like this and then criticizes B-17 for "false hope" is surely a hypocrite of the worst kind.

IS SATAN BEHIND THE ANTI-LAETRILE CAMPAIGN?

We now come to the most controversial section of this book. I realize full well the anger that I will bring down upon myself for the things I am about to write. Nevertheless, I feel that these things *must* be said. I am not a rabble-rouser and I am not the kind of person who is always looking for a fight. Just the opposite. All my life I have avoided fighting. But now I am getting my anger stirred up at the devil. I believe there is clear evidence that Satan is behind the anti-Laetrile campaign. I want to make it clear that I am not the kind of preacher who is always accusing others of being full of the devil just because their opinions conflict with mine. No, I deplore that sort of thing. I don't think we should blame all error and all sin on the devil. Certainly it is possible for men to err and even to sin purely on the basis of natural human weakness. So I am not suggesting that the devil is behind the opposition just to be harsh on my opponents. That's not it at all. In fact I feel quite sure that many of the opposition *think* they are doing right, and most of them certainly would not knowingly work for the devil. But God's Word says that Satan is a deceiver. He fools people into working for him when they do not realize it.

I have come to a firm conviction that Satan, the arch-enemy of God, is strongly involved in the anti-Laetrile campaign. I have not come to this conclusion suddenly or rashly. On the contrary, the conviction has developed slowly over the years as I have learned more about Satan and more about cancer. For almost thirty years I have taught courses on Satan in Bible institutes and colleges, so I am somewhat aware of his methods. And for about seven years I have carefully studied the Laetrile controversy. So I have had ample opportunity to give serious thought to this problem. The more I study the matter, the more evidence I see that the devil hates any natural cancer treatment and is working behind the scenes to stop its use.

Of course there are also some strictly human reasons for opposing any natural cancer therapy. I will mention here the most obvious ones. Men of this world could oppose B-17 for these reasons, without any help from the devil.

Inertia. The natural tendency is to maintain the status quo. When men have a comfortable system going, they naturally resist having it disturbed.

Erroneous Assumptions. It is easy to assume that nothing in nature could combat cancer. But we have shown before that this is an atheistic assumption.

Over-Confidence. Many physicians have an abnormal confidence that their group can handle the cancer problem without any help from chemists, from nature, from outside researchers, from "religious meddlers," and perhaps even from God.

Pride. It would be a severe blow to the pride of organized medicine if the cancer problem should be solved by a simple vitamin.

Economics. A considerable portion of the physician's training is in the field of medical economics. He is educated in methods of protecting his economic welfare. The evidence indicates that medical societies do not exist to protect the health of the patients, but to protect the income of the physicians. It has often been pointed out that the cancer industry has become so large that today there are more people making a living from cancer than are dying from it. Some students of economics have stated that if the cancer problem is suddenly solved it will seriously disturb the American economy. We will give proof later that there are powerful forces in our land that would rather see thousands die of cancer than see what they consider an economic disaster. If the reader cares to do further research, he will find documentary proof of an international drug cartel that controls a monopoly of the cancer industry in several books listed in the reading list at the end of this book.

Fear. There are many physicians and government agents that first began their B-17 opposition sincerely. Since then they have seen evidence that perhaps they were wrong. But what are they going to do now? It could be dangerous to admit error. Let's imagine a typical case. A man sees his child suffering with cancer. He hears of vitamin B-17 therapy and seeks to try it. He is blocked by some physician or government agent. He watches his loved one suffer the cutting, burning, and poisoning of the "approved" therapies. Finally the patient is given up to die an agonizing death. Then suppose the father learns that the "approved" treatments were of no value and that B-17 really does control cancer. What will he do? One day this is going to happen and no doubt some violent revenge will fall on the heads of those who blocked B-17 therapy. We do not condone violence in any circumstances, but we can certainly understand how a man in this situation could be overcome with rage and could attack the one whom he feels is responsible for the needless suffering and death of his loved one. Many persons who have interfered with B-17 therapy now realize they are wrong, but they are afraid. They are trying to postpone for a while longer the inevitable day when their enormous wrong is brought to light.

When vitamin B-17 is finally approved and comes into full public knowledge, there will be some serious repercussions. As the old saying goes, "some heads will roll." Government agents will be fired. Doctors will lose their practices. Judges who made anti-Laetrile rulings will be humiliated. The entire American people will lose confidence in the government agencies and medical societies that were supposedly looking out for their health. The anti-Laetrile forces know all this, and they are running scared. Even the sincere men who first thought they were right and now see they are wrong are scared and don't know what to do. Certainly the fear of reprisal is one influence that delays the full approval of vitamin B-17.

So much for the purely human reasons for opposing natural cancer remedies. Let's get down to the main subject at hand. What evidence is there that there may be more than human powers involved in the anti-Laetrile campaign? Is Satan at work in this matter? Hundreds and perhaps thousands of informed Christians believe that he is. I believe Satan is behind the opposition because of the following evidence:

Satan Always Opposes God's Way. We have already shown abundant evidence that God put B-17 in nature in all parts of the world. We have explained the chemical wonders by which B-17 kills malignant cells and nourishes non-malignant cells. This is clearly a plan of God's. It is Satan's purpose to work against God. It is logical to assume that the devil would want to interfere with this life-saving plan of God's. Just as God is life, so Satan has the power of death (Heb. 2:14). It is to his advantage to have people die.

The Opposition Is So Illogical. The inconsistency and absurdity of the anti-Laetrile campaign is so great that it is hard to believe that intelligent human beings could be this illogical without supernatural help. These same people are not that illogical in other areas of thought. For example, hundreds of known poisons are permitted in our food processing, but B-17 must not be used. All currently approved chemical agents for cancer therapy are admittedly poisonous, but harmless B-17 cannot be used. Cigarettes have been proved beyond question to be a contributing factor in lung cancer. But all the government has done about it is to have an ineffective warning printed on the package. But harmless B-17 is totally banned! Do you see any logic in that? Men do not normally think as stupidly as that. The Bible teaches that the devil blinds men's minds. It would be hard for us to explain how intelligent men can be so inconsistent unless Satan is helping to blind their minds!

The American Cancer Society receives approximately 100 million dollars annually in donations for cancer research. Only about half of this is spent on their futile research methods. The other half is spent on salaries and on anti-Laetrile propaganda. They have consistently refused to test B-17. Is this logical?

Government agencies are opposing B-17 more than marijuana. One day recently a man was arrested for bringing a few ounces of B-17 (which is nothing more than de-fatted apricot kernels) across the border. That same day another man was arrested for bringing 2½ pounds of dangerous marijuana across the border. The apricot smuggler's bond was set at $50,000 (higher than a murderer's bond) and he spent eight days in jail. The dope smuggler did not have to pay bond and was released on his own recognizance. Let's face it, many agencies of our government don't care how much poisonous dope is brought into this country. But they are determined to to let in health-giving substances that might reduce the income of the cancer industry. Is this logical? The devil is behind this!

The Opposition Is So Unfair. Nothing could be more unfair than the current methods being used to discredit B-17. For example, it is often claimed that this vitamin has not been sufficiently researched, yet our existing laws practically prevent such research. If you were a cancer researcher, and you were about to prove a natural substance to be effective in treating cancer, and if you knew a jail cell awaited you at the end of your research, would you continue? Is this fair?

Every year thousands of patients go through the usual routine of surgery, radiation, and chemotherapy and are then given up as hopeless. They are sent home to die. In this state of near-death they turn to Laetrile as a last resort, but it is too late. When they die, the anti-Laetrile forces point to this as proof that Laetrile is a failure. Why do they not point to this as proof of orthodox therapy failure? Is this fair?

Physicians who are dedicated enough and courageous enough to use B-17 are immediately branded as "quacks." They are in danger of losing their licenses. They may lose their hospital privileges. They can even go to jail. They are assumed guilty without a trial. A real trial would include a scientific investigation of the effectiveness of the treatment, but this is never done. Is this fair? Men are not normally this unfair. It would appear that the devil is involved in any campaign as unfair and vicious as this.

The Opposition Is Based on Falsehood. Truth and falsehood are profound spiritual principles. Jesus Christ is "the truth" (John 14:6). Conversely Satan is the one who speaks "the lie" (John 8:44, Greek). So truth and falsehood are identified with two persons, Christ and Satan. All truth is from God, and serves the purposes of God. Not just truth in the religious realm, but all truth. Likewise all lies serve the purposes of Satan. Not just religious lies, but all lies. The medieval lies about the earth and the sun were not exactly religious lies; they were scientific lies. Nevertheless it seems clear that Satan used those lies to dishonor God and to destroy some very great men. So we need to realize that lies in any field of human experience can serve the purposes of the devil.

It is not my intention to accuse any human being of lying, for I do not have the proof in my possession. But I do know that many lies are being told to prevent the use of vitamin B-17. In some cases the persons who make these statements may *think* they are telling the truth. But the statements are still lies. Perhaps Satan started the lies and possibly men repeat them thinking them to be true. But they are still lies serving the purposes of the devil.

Here is an example of a falsehood commonly used to scare people away from B-17. The charge is made that B-17 is "illegal." This is often an attempt to make the public think it is illegal to manufacture, sell, or use the substance for any purpose in any state. This is deception. As has been explained before, it is illegal in California and a few other states for doctors to use it as a cancer specific. But it is not illegal in any state to use it for general nutritional purposes.

The anti-Laetrile forces constantly prove their untruthfulness by contradicting themselves. First they say that B-17 is useless because there is no way to release the cyanide from it. Then they say B-17 should be banned because it will release cyanide which may be toxic! Again they contradict themselves when they say B-17 should not be used because it has not been tested, then they say B-17 has been tested and found useless. Government agents have gone on record saying that there is not a shred of evidence indicating that B-17 has any anti-cancer value. Dr. Dean Burk, internationally famous former head of the cytochemistry division of the National Cancer Institute, says publicly that they are liars. He has stated frequently on radio and on television that they are liars, and he has named names. He has gone on record, in print, naming laboratory research projects here and abroad that have found positive results using B-17.

The Mexican government has reportedly sent records of 1200 patients successfully treated with B-17 to the United States FDA. Yet the FDA claims they have not seen a "shred of evidence." Are they lying?

Dr. Krebs has publicly accused the FDA of deliberate lies and deception. He has stated vehemently that the FDA is carrying on a deliberate, premeditated plan to deceive the American public about the safety and effectiveness of B-17. George Kell, the highly successful Laetrile defense attorney who has rarely lost such a case, has publicly stated the same thing. All of these men have referred to specific persons and specific statements (see the reading list for details). Since none of these men have been sued for libel, we must conclude that they have abundant proof of their accusations.

Another example of lying is the charge that only quacks use B-17. We have already given the names of some of the world's most eminent scientists who use B-17. One more falsehood is the charge that Laetrile promoters are making vast profits off of cancer victims. The fact is that Laetrile can be purchased in this country for 10% above the price established by the government of Mexico. Compare this with a commonly-used orthodox drug, such as Valium, which sells in this country for over 100,000 times the cost at the factory in Sweden. Christians should not be deceived by such false accusations.

The entire anti-Laetrile campaign reeks of falsehoods. Truth is slandered, information is obscured, and every conceivable device is used to keep the truth from being known.

Jesus said, "Ye shall know the truth, and the truth shall make you free" (John 8:32). Why do the anti-Laetrile forces try to keep American cancer patients from learning about Laetrile? Even if the substance had very little value, there is no excuse for trying to hide the truth. Who hates the truth? The devil does!

The Opposition Is Unconstitutional. The Constitution of the United States is a very special document. This nation is the first in history to be founded specifically to obtain Christian freedom, and the Constitution is the document to guarantee that freedom. The Constitution, though imperfect, is based strongly on Bible principles. The problem with our Constitution is not with the way it is written, but rather the way it is administered. Many citizens think that the Constitution will automatically protect their rights. Nothing could be further from the truth. The Constitution never did automatically protect anyone. Let me illustrate. It is traditional in this country for the Congress to vaguely define the powers of any new agency they create. It is also traditional that any government agency will push its powers to the limit and beyond the limits prescribed by Congress. It is almost routine for government bureaucrats to go beyond their designated powers and to violate the constitutional rights of citizens. Does the Constitution then automatically protect that citizen? Of course not! The citizen must secure legal assistance and file his complaint in court for relief. But it will cost him plenty in time and money to get the rights guaranteed to him by the Constitution.

There have already been several cases where government agents have arrested and jailed physicians for using B-17 as a nutritional supplement. In several such cases the courts have found that the arrest was unconstitutional. That means that the agents were law-breakers and that the arrested physician was a good, law-abiding citizen. In such a case the law-breaking officials cannot be punished for their crime. But the physician has had his name slandered and still has a police record. You see, the bureaucrats have everything to gain and nothing to lose by these unconstitutional methods!

The unconstitutional nature of the FDA's Laetrile opposition can be shown in another way. Our Constitution guarantees equal protection under the law for all citizens. Now let's see if we have that equal protection. I have a neighbor who has diabetes, another with arthritis, another with emphysema. The U.S. Food and Drug Administration will allow these patients to use any substance they want as long as the patient and the doctor agree on it. They can even use deadly narcotics, like morphine, if they want to do so. But I am a cancer patient, and the FDA would prevent me and my physician from using B-17 if they could. This clearly violates our constitutional principle of equal treatment to all. I challenge anyone to give logical explanation showing that it does not.

We hear a lot of talk these days about minorities being mistreated. All such mistreatment is bad of course. But I am a member of the most cruelly mistreated minority in America, for I am a cancer patient. And if certain government agencies and medical authorities have their way, one thousand of us each day will be sentenced to die a slow and agonizing death, forbidden to use the relief that God has given us. I defy anyone to find a more mistreated minority group! This is discrimination of the worst kind. The educational and employment discrimination we hear so much about is nothing compared to the ruthless slaughter of 1,000 helpless victims every day! The reading list will show documented proof that this unconstitutional discrimination is for the purpose of protecting a cancer monopoly. Do you doubt that Satan is behind this monstrous evil?

The Opposition Is Cruel and Vicious. We have already pointed to some cruelties. But there are yet more. Notice how cruel this is. Years ago, Dr. Krebs was tried and convicted as a result of his wonderful discovery of B-17. We believe this conviction was false, unconstitutional, and clearly against the will of God. But now government agencies point to this jail sentence as "proof" that Krebs is a "quack." How cruel can you get? The Apostle Paul was imprisoned for preaching the gospel of Jesus Christ. His enemies then pointed to his prison record as "proof" that he was a fake. You see, times have not changed. The devil still uses the same methods today that he used long ago.

The opposition is cruel because they block research and testing. This means they do not want the truth. The Bible makes clear that Satan hates truth. Honest men have nothing to fear from scientific research and the full exposure of truth.

The worst cruelty of all is this. The American Medical Association wants Laetrile banned because it may cause patients to neglect surgery or other "approved" methods. Let's see if that claim is sincere. Thousands of patients have already gone through the gauntlet of cutting, burning, and poisoning and have been given up as hopeless. The doctors have said in effect, "Go home and die, we cannot hlep you." Now these patients are no longer candidates for the usual therapies. Is there any reason to withhold B-17 from them? Most patients find it gives great relief from cancer pain. Since the danger of the patient neglecting surgery is no longer an issue, he can have his B-17 now, can't he? NO! *He is still forbidden to have B-17*. The AMA and the FDA are still determined that the physician must not use B-17 to relieve the agony of a dying person. Why not? They admit it will do no harm.

Why not indeed? This is indescribably cruel. There is only one possible reason why anyone would deny a harmless relief to a dying person. Here it is. There is a danger that some of these dying persons might recover because of the B-17. This would never do, because it would prove to the world in a very dramatic way that Laetrile really does work after all! Have you ever seen such cruelty? Do you doubt that it is inspired by the devil?

At this point I know that some good naive Americans are going to say that they cannot believe that any Americans would let other Americans die just in order to make money. *Don't be simple-minded!* It has been going on right before our eyes for years. When our boys were dying in Vietnam, who do you think manufactured the weapons to kill them? It is a widely known fact that American businessmen sold weapons to European nations who in turn sold them to North Vietnam to be used to kill our boys. And the businessmen knew where they were going! Don't try to tell me that industry will not let thousands die in order to make profits! Let's wake up to reality. Do you still doubt Satan?

There Is a Conspiracy Against Laetrile. Thousands of Americans believe there is a powerfully organized conspiracy to keep B-17 and all other natural cancer remedies off the market. Of course the "authorities" ridicule this idea as the ravings of a paranoid mind. Well, let's just see if this is the case. Let's see if any intelligent and competent people believe there is a conspiracy.

In 1953, a congressional investigation of the cancer situation was begun. Senator Tobey, Chairman of the Interstate and Foreign Commerce Committee, appointed Benedict B. Fitzgerald of the Department of Justice to conduct the investigation. On August 11, 1953, Mr. Fitzgerald filed a report with the committee which read in part:

> Is there any dispute among recognized medical scientists in America and elsewhere in the world on the use of radium and X-ray therapy in the treatment of cancer? The answer is definitely Yes: there is a division of opinion on the use of radium and X-ray. Both agencies are destructive, not constructive. In the alleged destruction of the abnormal, outlaw, or cancer cells, both X-ray and radium destroy normal tissue and normal cells. Recognized medical authorities in America and elsewhere state positvely that X-ray therapy can cause cancer in, and of, itself. Documented cases are available.
>
> Accordingly, we should determine whether existing agencies, both public and private, are engaged, and have pursued a policy of harassment, ridicule, slander and libelous attacks on others sincerely engaged in stamping out this curse of mankind. Have

medical associations through their officers, agents, servants, and employees engaged in this practice? My investigation to date should convince this committee that a conspiracy does exist to stop the free flow and use of drugs in interstate commerce which allegedly have solid therapeutic value. Public and private funds have been thrown around like confetti to close up and destroy clinics and hospitals and scientific laboratories which do not conform to the viewpoint of medical associations.

In his complete and lengthy report, Mr. Fitzgerald stated that the American Medical Association and other groups were deliberately obstructing unorthodox cancer treatments. Senator Tobey died shortly thereafter, and the investigation was stopped.

How does the conspiracy work in practice? How can government bureaus destroy a physician who uses natural cancer therapies? There is a very simple and effective method. It was used to destroy Dr. Koch, Dr. Gerson, Dr. Ivy, Dr. Hoxsey, and others. It can destroy any man, even though he has violated no law. Here is how it works. One government bureau after another throws its big legal guns against the physician. He is dragged into court time and time again. In nearly every case the jury finds the physician innocent of any wrongdoing. Is he now free? By no means! He has been out tens of thousands of dollars in legal fees. He has been kept so busy with his legal defense that he has had to neglect his practice. His reputation has been smeared in the papers. He has been harassed and worried until he is a nervous wreck. But it is not over! Soon another government agency drags him into court again. More expense! More slander! More worry! And the bureaucrats can keep this up forever because they have unlimited taxpayers' money to spend on this prosecution. They know that if they keep this up long enough that the physician will finally be destroyed.

Notice that in this type of harassment it matters not that the physician is innocent. It matters not that the bureaucrats cannot get a conviction. In fact, they often realize they don't have a case and there is no chance of a conviction. But the process of slowly grinding the doctor to bits goes on relentlessly until he is destroyed. Too many of us Americans have imagined that the courts protect a man from false charges. Courts can find a man innocent, but there is no court that protects a man from such repeated harassment by an endless number of government agencies. Such agencies have the "right" to bring charges as often as they wish, until the physician is destroyed. One great cancer researcher after another has been destroyed by this extra-legal method. Several Laetrile physicians in California are now undergoing such organized persecution. Even though exonerated again and again in the courts, the juggernaut of conspired persecution goes on. It is important that Christians pray for these great dedicated men so they will not be destroyed by the enemies of truth.

The Bible refers frequently to conspiracies. In every case there is a clear suggestion that enormous evil is behind the conspiracy. Jesus Christ was crucified because of a conspiracy. The record indicates a clear conspiracy to deny cancer patients in this country access to all natural cancer treatments. Can you still doubt that Satan is involved in this dirty business?

Christians Are the Group Most Concerned About Laetrile. I certainly do not wish to imply that everyone who favors B-17 is a Christian and everyone who opposes B-17 is a non-Christian. By no means! A person becomes a Christian by repenting of his sins and trusting in the atoning sacrifice of Christ to pay for those sins. But in my experience I have noticed a definite pattern in this controversy. I have discussed the Laetrile controversy with hundreds of persons. I have noticed that every Bible-believing Christian I have talked to quickly takes a positive attitude toward B-17. They favor it because it is natural and God-given. They favor freeing it on grounds of fairness, even though they may not be sure of its value. They can understand that an evil conspiracy could be behind the opposition because this is consistent with Biblical teachings and historical experience. I have received hundreds of telephone calls from strangers who wanted further information about B-17. Almost always the caller is a deeply religious person.

On the other hand, I am thinking of one man whom I told about the B-17 controversy. He immediately rejected the idea. Why? He told me that men were naturally good and would never be guilty of such an evil. What was his problem? He did not believe the Bible. He did not accept the Biblical teaching that men have sinful hearts and are capable of great wickedness. I have attended many conventions where B-17 and other natural cancer treatments were being acvocated. In every case most of the speakers and most of the delegates were either genuine Christians or at least persons with a deep regard for the goodness of God in creation.

It Is Religious Discrimination. Our Constitution forbids the favoring of one religious group over another, yet there are agencies of our government, and even courts, that consistently violate this principle. There are Indian tribes in America that are allowed to use dangerous narcotics even though they are properly forbidden by law. Why are they allowed this special privilege? These tribes claim that their religious beliefs require the use of these narcotics. But there are thousands of Christians who firmly believe, on the basis of good evidence, that God put B-17 in our environment for the prevention of cancer. They also believe, with good reason, that it is their religious responsibility to care for the body which is the temple of the Holy Spirit. But government agencies seek to deny them this opportunity. Will someone please explain why Indians may use a dangerous drug for religious reasons but Christians may not use a harmless food for religious reasons? Now are you still in favor of banning B-17? What happened to your respect for constitutional equality?

All this clear evidence should make us consider strongly the probability that Satan himself is behind the conspiracy to outlaw vitamin B-17. If someone doesn't think so, then I would like to hear a better explanation for this whole dirty mess!

THE PROPER ROLE OF GOVERNMENT

This whole stinking legal mess makes it necessary for us to examine the proper role of government. Why did God establish human government anyway? Was it His intention for government to set up an endless list of bureaus to control every detail of human life? *Absolutely Not!* Human government was established by God in Genesis 9:5-6. The purpose of government was plainly stated to be the punishment of violent offenders. God's intended role of government is to discourage violent crime, not to regulate every detail of life! Enormous evil has resulted when government has departed from its proper role and tried to play god instead.

Christians are to obey government, but they are also to be aware and greatly concerned when government steps out of its God-given role. Does the reader recall the details of the Dred Scott case, when the Supreme Court ruled that a black man was not entitled to the equal protection of the law that the Constitution guaranteed to every man? On what grounds? The court ruled that while a black man did have a brain and a heart, he was nevertheless not a human being! Now, I ask the reader, did that make it so, just because the Supreme Court said so? You see, the government is not God, and when government gets out of its God-given assignment and tries to dictate every detail of human life, great evil results. This is where the devil gets in.

The Bible warns that the dictatorial powers of centralized government will become worse and worse in the last days. This oppressive power will finally culminate in a world dictator, commonly called the Antichrist, who will rule the world by the power of Satan. Every Christian who understands Bible prophecy is concerned that the trend is already moving toward the Antichrist. Christians must be concerned when government begins moving in the direction of dictatorship and the destruction of human freedoms. The informed Christian will be opposed to all government and medical society interference with B-17. The patient and doctor should have the freedom to use this therapy if they desire. Even if a Christian does not believe B-17 is effective, he still should support this freedom of choice on grounds of fairness and equality.

Legal interference with natural cancer therapies is wrong. It is immoral. It is ungodly. Every Christian should be deeply concerned about it, and we should pray earnestly that the day will soon come when God's relief for human misery will no longer be "illegal."

Learning this awful principle has been somewhat of a shock. But since it is "illegal" for God to relieve cancer misery, I am glad that I became aware of it. Learning of this awful situation has enabled me to give encouragement and help to many trapped cancer victims. It has been worth having cancer myself to be able to help others who are caught in this awful trap. So again, I can thank God for cancer!

"In every thing give thanks"
(1 Thessalonians 5:18)

I can thank God for cancer, for it caused me to see this practical life-saving truth—

PRINCIPLE NO. 10: WE CAN COOPERATE WITH GOD ANYWAY

Many cancer victims are paralyzed into inaction when they hear the propaganda that B-17 is "illegal." As we have seen, this charge is partly true but mostly false. But the cancer patient often doesn't know the whole truth, so he is scared away by the false propaganda. Especially if he is a Christian, he wants to obey the law and so he is afraid to try amygdalin therapy. It is most unfortunate that unscrupulous propagandists will take advantage of the high morality of many cancer victims to deceive them into inaction. I have personally known of more than one dying Christian who could have obtained pain relief and possibly could have recovered by the use of B-17. Yet they declined to do so because they had heard that it was "illegal." It is difficult to conceive of anything more tragic than this.

This places the cancer patient between the two horns of the dilemma. On the one hand, it is his Christian duty to care for his body, the temple of the Holy Spirit. On the other hand it is his duty to obey the laws of his country. How can he do both? What can he do when caught in this web of legal confusion? How can he protect himself from this cruel and oppressive situation? Most important, how can he find the will of God when he apparently has two conflicting moral duties? There is always a way out. God will guide his child through the darkest night of trial.

> There hath no temptation [trial] taken you but such as is common to man: but God is faithful, who will not suffer you to be tempted above that ye are able; but will with the temptation also make a way to escape, that ye may be able to bear it. (1 Cor. 10:13)

> While we are praying for God to make a way of escape, we must realize that we have a

responsibility ourselves. Humanly speaking, the cancer victim's only hope is education. He must learn all he can about the legal, medical, and nutritional aspects of this problem. That's why you are reading this book. And that's why you must continue reading from the list given at the end and from other sources as well. The admonition of the Lord Jesus Christ is especially appropriate here, "Be wise as serpents, and harmless as doves" (Matt. 10:16). In these terrible circumstances, wisdom can save your life—so learn!

LEARN THE TRUTH ABOUT METABOLIC THERAPY

By metabolic therapy we mean the control of the body chemistry by means of vitamins, minerals, enzymes, proteins, and other food factors so that the body can heal itself. Such chronic diseases as cancer, arthritis, and diabetes are problems of the body metabolism, and if they are to be controlled it must be by correcting that metabolism.

For the cancer patient, the most important single metabolic substance seems to be vitamin B-17. But this must not be thought of as a miracle drug that "cures" everyone who uses it. Cancer control, like the control of any chronic metabolic disease, requires the teamwork of many metabolic substances. So B-17 is not something magic, but it is the most important member of the cancer-fighting team. The cancer patient who uses B-17 only, and does not use the other vitamins and enzymes and does not follow the recommended diet, can expect poor results. On the other hand, the patient who gets on the complete metabolic program, including vitamin B-17, and gets on it early enough can usually expect good results.

SOME CASE HISTORIES

To illustrate the good results that might be obtained, let me mention some case histories from my own observation. These are not professional case histories, but merely the observations of a layman. Several of these patients were personal friends of mine. Others were close relatives of my personal friends. In every case, I had opportunity to know the circumstances.

R. D., a 14 year old boy in Dallas, Texas, developed a brain tumor in 1967. The surgeons found that so much of the brain was involved that it was impossible to remove all of the tumor. The prediction was that the tumor would inevitably grow again and that the patient could not live longer than six months. Soon after this, the patient was placed on vitamin B-17 and other nutritional factors. After eight and one half years there has been no reappearance of the malignancy.

Mr. B. B., of Dallas County, Texas, developed lung cancer in 1972, and part of one lung was removed. Two years later, ten more lung tumors were discovered by X-ray. The prediction was that he could only survive a matter of months. The patient was placed on chemotherapy. He also began taking B-17, but did not inform his physician about this. The physician expressed surprise that the tumors were disappearing. In spite of shrinking tumors, the patient was very ill and his condition continued to deteriorate. After several weeks in the hospital in a near-death condition, he requested to go home so that he could discontinue the chemotherapy and resume his B-17. I later visited him in his home and he told me he no longer had any pain. He told me that he "would rather die tomorrow than have another shot of chemotherapy." He suffered no more pain for the remaining days of his life.

Mrs. D. T., age 56, of Canton, Texas, had a tumor on her head in 1969 which was diagnosed as malignant. Extensive radiation was required to reduce the tumor. One year later the malignancy reappeared, this time in the roof of the mouth. Again prolonged radiation was needed to reduce the swelling. In 1973, the malignancy returned again. This time the diagnosis was much more serious. The malignancy was now general and widespread, involving the lymphatic system and the bone marrow. The patient was informed that her life expectancy was only two years, but that prolonged chemotherapy might extend this "if it works." Chemotherapy was begun, resulting in severe sickness, pain, and loss of hair. Following a church service, the patient approached me and asked me to pray for her. She told me that she would rather die than have another chemotherapy treatment. Her feeling was that if she was going to die, she would rather die naturally and with dignity than be destroyed by man-made poisons. At this time she had never heard of B-17 or any natural therapy. She refused further chemotherapy and in early 1974 began metabolic therapy, including vitamin B-17. At this writing, two years later, she has had no further "approved" therapy and is living a normal active life, feeling better than she has in years. She recently informed me that she had returned to the same major Dallas hospital where, in 1973, she was pronounced terminal. But this time she went in only for a check up. The doctors told her they could find no trace of cancer!

Mr. E. C., of Atlanta, Texas, suffered severe back pains of unknown origin, and for over a year was unable to sleep on his back. The appearance of a tumor on the head in 1974 led to a physical examination, at which time lung cancer was discovered. He was told that he could live only a few months. At this time he was too sick to work. Amygdalin treatment was begun, and after the third injection his back pain was gone and he was able to sleep on his back. He was also able to return to work. He did not inform his original physician of the B-17 treatment. When he returned to a world famous cancer hospital in Houston, Texas, the doctors expressed surprise that the tumor on his head had diminished in size. They said they had never seen this type of tumor shirnk before. The patient continued to have considerable difficulty, but was able to work most of the time as long as he remained on his metabolic program.

Mr. H. E., of Dallas, Texas, age 72, developed cancer of the tongue, mouth, and neck in 1972. For two years he underwent repeated treatments with radioactive cobalt. He suffered severe burns and extreme sickness. The malignancy was reduced some but remained largely resistant to the radiation. During the course of treatment his weight dropped from 220 lbs. to 145 lbs. In June of 1974, he was completely unable to work and his condition was deteriorating rapidly. It was apparent that the end was drawing near. The patient was so sick of the radiation misery that he told his family that he would rather die than have another treatment. At this time his son tried to persuade him to try B-17. He had no confidence at all in it but began the treatment just to please his son. At this writing, a year and a half later, Mr. E. is 75 years old and works full time every day. He is a carpenter and regularly climbs on top of the roof. He is in excellent condition for a man of his age.

Dr. M. F., a Dallas, Texas, dentist, developed cancer of the tongue in 1974. In December of that year, surgeons planned to remove part of his tongue. This he refused, and began a program of metabolic therapy, including vitamin B-17. Within a few months the tongue healed completely. The patient is continuing his metabolic program to prevent recurrence. He states that his health and vigor are now much better than before he developed cancer.

Dr. G. M., a Dallas, Texas, chiropractor, age 49, suffered from rectal polyps and bleeding for many years. In early 1975, his condition was diagnosed as squamos cell carcinoma of the rectum. A colostomy was scheduled, but the patient declined to have it performed. Further examination indicated a metastasis to the left kidney. The patient obtained the services of another surgeon who agreed to omit the colostomy and to remove only some small areas of cancerous tissue. Prior to this surgery he began a program of metabolic therapy including vitamin B-17. No orthodox treatment was given for the diseased kidney. Many months later, on the same day that I was writing this paragraph, the patient called me on the telephone to tell me how happy he was over his progress. He says he feels fine and that two prominent physicians, one in America and one in a foreign country, have expressed the opinion that his malignancy is now under control.

Mr. J. S., of Richardson, Texas, developed cancer of the throat in 1975. Doctors removed all of his teeth to enable them to get the radiation equipment down into his throat. The radiation burned his throat so severely that he was unable to swallow. Patient had heard of B-17 but had declined to use it. As a last resort he began B-17 therapy. To his doctor's dismay, he refused further radiation. Within three weeks he was feeling fine and was rejoicing over the wonders of metabolic therapy.

To this list I could add my own case. I have had obvious malignant symptoms since 1967. In 1969, I was scheduled for a permanent colostomy. The operating room already had me down for an appointment, but I have postponed this procedure for almost seven years. Not only have I brought the malignancy under control by amygdalin therapy, but my general health is much better today than seven years ago.

It is important for the cancer victim to be convinced of the merit of B-17. If he begins the program merely as an experiment, he may quickly discontinue it because of lack of self-discipline or because of the cost factor. Assurance of B-17 effectiveness can be gained by reading other case histories, many of which are given in the books on the reading list. Most of these are from professional sources. Anyone who really wants to know what B-17 is doing can find out. The literature on the subject is abundant.

BEWARE OF THE CANCER TRAP!

Many cancer patients, after years of surgery, radiation, and chemotherapy, express the feeling that they have been caught in a trap. They feel that they have been cast on an assembly line, where surgery leads inevitably to radiation, and in turn radiation leads inevitably to chemotherapy, and in turn chemotherapy leads inevitably to general bodily deterioration and finally death. They complain because it seems that the whole assembly line is preplanned. They also are bitter because they seem to have no choice in the matter. They feel trapped.

The reader should not misunderstand this discussion. I am not stating my own opinion of the currently used therapies, but merely referring to the fact that a great many patients do feel trapped. I am not implying that no one should ever have these treatments I have mentioned. I never advise anyone to use or not to use the so-called orthodox treatments. But I do contend that every patient should be thoroughly informed so that he can make an intelligent choice. So many persons who have chosen the route of approved therapy later feel that they were rushed into it because of fear, pressure, and ignorance.

Perhaps the reader is asking, "Well, just what do you believe about orthodox cancer treatments?" I accept the opinions of the many internationally famous scientists who understand both orthodox therapies and metabolic therapy. In general, they believe that surgery does not cure cancer and that it should be employed only as a last resort to relieve a blockage or something of that nature. They believe that radiation sometimes helps skin cancer but is practically useless and possibly very harmful in internal cancer. They believe that certain forms of chemotherapy applied locally to skin cancer are sometimes helpful. They believe that chemotherapy used internally is deadly poisonous and is likely to do more harm than good. Generally speaking then, the usual therapies are at best a gamble. They may help, but almost certainly they will do harm. The worst part of all is this: all three of these types of therapy can actually spread cancer! How? There are two ways: they all injure the body, and cancer usually starts and spreads where there is injury; and they all destroy the disease-fighting mechanism that God has placed in the body. Is it right for a Christian to destroy God's disease-fighting mechanism and to replace it with a man-made system of doubtful value?

The reader should understand that this is not necessarily a criticism of your own personal physician. Most doctors are honest and dedicated men. The criticism should be directed at an international drug and industrial cartel that controls the cancer monopoly. The practicing physician only knows what the schools and medical journals tell him, and these are controlled by the monopoly. A large number of physicians are now becoming disillusioned with current therapies. In frustration they are exclaiming, "They've got to give us something better than this to fight cancer!"

More and more people are becoming aware of the cancer trap. More and more are waking up to the reality that the cancer monopoly has looked upon the patient as expendable merchandise, a source of income to be exploited. The average cancer patient is worth $15,000 to the cancer industry. And he usually has insurance. The cancer industry cannot afford to let this insurance money go to waste!

So don't get caught in the cancer trap! If you have surgery, know what you are doing. Know that it is necessary. Make the decision yourself. Don't let fear tactics stampede you into getting on the assembly line. Best of all, try to find a physician who understands metabolic therapy. If he believes surgery necessary, he will perform or recommend the least possible cutting. He will not damage the body unnecessarily. And he certainly is not likely to cast you on the assembly line. Information will be given later on locating such a physician.

UNDERSTAND THE RELATION OF THE CHRISTIAN TO THE LAW

Many cancer patients have suffered and died

needlessly because of confusion about their legal responsibilities. Many could have been saved by B-17, but declined to use it because someone scared them with the word *illegal*. They did not realize that they could have used this natural treatment without violating any legal, moral, or Biblical principle. In fact, once the truth is understood, the patient will probably conclude that it is morally wrong not to use B-17.

The Christian's relationship to human law is not simple, because of the enormously complex and sometimes contradictory nature of human law. Christian scholars have struggled with these complex problems for many centuries, and much has been written on the subject. It is impossible to give an exact answer in advance for every legal question that a person may face, but the careful student of the Word of God will find certain basic principles clearly established.

God Judges the Motive. Of course a person must not excuse an obvious wrong by claiming a noble motive. But in a situation where there are conflicting principles and the right is difficult to determine, the motive of the heart is basic. God does not judge actions as such, but He judges the heart. Purely selfish motives will bring on the judgment of a holy God. For example, one who brings apricot seeds across the border in order to survive is not the same as one who brings apricot seeds across the border in order to extract excessive profits from cancer victims.

Even human courts recognize motive as basic in determining guilt.

Human Laws Are to Be Obeyed Wherever Possible. The principle of human government is established by God Himself. He who rebels against human law is rebelling against God (Rom. 13:1-2), the one exception being when one has to disobey man's law in order to obey God. Christians have a special reason for being submissive to law, and that is to protect their testimony and influence for Jesus Christ. Man's law should never be resisted for shallow or selfish reasons.

God's Law Is Supreme Over All Laws. In case a human law clearly contradicts God's law, then God's law must prevail. The apostles of Jesus Christ refused to obey man's law when they were ordered not to speak of Jesus Christ (Acts 4:18-20). Human law contradicted God's law during the Spanish Inquisition when thousands of persons were burned at the stake for claiming that Christ alone could forgive sins. It was the Christian's duty to rebel against that human law. Human law opposed the law of God under Hitler when millions of Jews were put to death "legally" for the crime of being Jews. It was the Christian's duty to resist that human law. Human law contradicted the divine law in the Dred Scott Case, when the U.S. Supreme Court ruled that Negroes were not human beings. It was the Christian's duty to oppose that human law. You see, the government is not God, and when it gets out of its proper sphere and tries to be God, then Christians must obey the true God, not the false one.

God's law teaches us to save human life wherever possible. If a human law condemns 1,000 innocent victims a day to die of cancer, and denies them a harmless, God-given relief, then the Christian must decide whether he will support God's law or man's.

The Highest American Law Is the Constitution. The American who desires to support the law in America frequently runs into trouble, for one law sometimes contradicts another law. Which one shall he support? This may not be simple. But it is fundamental to our system that all laws must conform to the Constitution. The Federal courts have ruled that when an unconstitutional law is enacted, that no one is obliged to obey it and no court or agency should enforce it. This is absolutely logical. Yet in practice there are serious problems. It is a fact of history that American states and cities often enact legislation that is later shown to be unconstitutional. Also, power-hungry government bureaucrats regularly issue their decrees that are later shown to be unconstitutional. It usually takes a long time for such a matter to be declared unconstitutional by the courts. But remember this, if it is finally declared to be unconstitutional, then it *was unconstitutional* before it was declared so by the courts. During that time then, those who conformed to such decrees were morally wrong and those who resisted were morally right. That can put a highly ethical person in a very difficult position. You see, knowing how to obey the law is not all that simple in our terribly complex legal environment.

Here is a case in point. Every physician for centuries has taken the Oath of Hippocrates, which states among other things that he will do all in his power to save the life of his patient. Courts have also ruled that this is his legal responsibility. But a California statute forbids doctors to treat cancer with God-given B-17. Here are two laws that conflict. Which one shall the physician obey? In time the absurd anti-Laetrile law will be ruled unconstitutional. Therefore it is unconstitutional now. What then is the duty of the physician right now?

Sometimes a person who makes a big pretense of obeying the law is just a petty coward with no moral character. In bowing to the unconstitutional decree of some power-hungry bureaucrat, he may actually be violating the highest law of our land and also the law of God Almighty! Thank God for those Christian doctors who have the character and conviction to put higher laws above lower laws. That's the kind of men that built this nation!

It Is Legal to Flee from Oppressive Rule. If a person cannot get legal treatment with B-17 in his own area then it is right for him to go where it is legal. To prove this, let us look at a case concerning the Lord Jesus Christ. The rulers of His land were conspiring to put Him to death. Since it was not time for Him to die, He left the country to preserve His life. This establishes a great moral principle. If a Christian finds his life threatened by cruel and oppressive government edicts, it is his Christian right and duty to go elsewhere. The Christian should not hesitate to go to a foreign country to receive Laetrile treatment if he desires to do so. However, as we shall show later, this is often not necessary. No person should have any guilty feelings about the use of B-17 merely because he may have heard rumors that it is "illegal." It is legal on both Biblical and constitutional grounds when properly used, as the next section shows.

UNDERSTAND THE CURRENT LEGAL STATUS OF B-17

We have already discussed many of the details of the legal situation. It will be necessary only to summarize the legal facts here. The cancer patient and other interested parties should have these facts clearly in mind so as to be able to refute erroneous statements they may hear concerning B-17's legality.
Personal Use of B-17 Is Legal in All States. This substance has been widely used for over 130 years to treat many conditions. It is recognized as a natural, non-toxic food substance and has never been regulated as far as

manufacture, sale, or use as a general nutritional substance.

Professional Nutritional Use of B-17 Is Legal in All States. Any doctor in America can legally use B-17 as a general nutritional or metabolic substance.

Professional Use of B-17 as a Specific Anti-Cancer Substance Is Forbidden in a Few States. California and a few other states forbid doctors to use B-17 specifically to treat cancer. But they define cancer as a "lump" or a "bump." But no Laetrile physician uses the substance to treat "lumps and bumps." They all use it along with other substances to treat the entire body. So even if the physician knows that the B-17 will control the cancer, he still is within the law because he is not treating "lumps and bumps." The FDA and their allies have consistently persecuted physicians for curing or relieving cancer with this harmless and effective substance. But in eleven lawsuits the courts have consistently ruled that the physicians are not violating any law because they are treating the whole body and not a "lump or bump."

The entire law has been ruled unconstitutional in lower courts. It may take a long time for the Supreme Court to make a final and nationwide ruling. In the meantime the bureaucrats don't care if it is unconstitutional. They will continue to harass the users of B-17 until forced by the courts to cease.

Rightly used then, any doctor or individual

can use B-17 with no fear of violating any legal or moral principle. His only problem is harassment from lawless bureaucrats.

OBSERVE THE BASIC PRINCIPLES OF NATURAL HEALTH

This book is written on the assumption that some of my readers will be totally uninformed in this vitally important area. Therefore the better informed reader will please forgive our repetition of these elementary principles.

Cancer patients often hope for some magic cure that will stop the disease quickly and easily. No such cure exists and no such cure will ever be found. Why? Because cancer is the result of a breakdown of the body metabolism. Normally there are many contributing factors working over a long period of time. If the malignancy is to be brought under control, then the cause must be removed. In order to restore proper metabolism, the patient will have to change his entire lifestyle. His eating habits must change. He must be willing to do much reading and study of the literature in this field. He may have to change his way of thinking, his emotional habits, and possibly even his environment. The patient who refuses to make these adjustments and hopes for a magic pill will probably wait in vain. Since cancer is the result of many years of wrong diet and wrong living, the patient must realize that his problem is due to his failure to cooperate with God, even though such failure may have been due to ignorance. If he is to recover, then he must begin to cooperate with God in all areas of his life, and this includes observing the principles of natural health.

A good place to start cooperating with nature is to start a compost heap and an organic garden. More and more Americans are learning how to grow their own delicious vegetables free from chemical fertilizers and poisonous insecticides. Information about organic gardening may be obtained from any health food store, most libraries, and many book stores.

The patient must become aware of the vast difference in natural foods (God-given) and processed foods (man-made). He must form the habit of being alert at all times to this distinction. If he insists on continuing his diet of processed foods, his recovery will be hindered in proportion to the amount of processed foods consumed.

The patient should become familiar with the services performed by the health food stores. At this point it is not my purpose to praise or to condemn health food stores. I would like to present what I believe is the proper attitude toward these places of business. First, I do not like to use the term *health foods,* for I think it is misleading. Not everything that is called *health food* is healthy, and not everything sold in supermarkets is unhealthy. I think it is better to think in terms of *natural* foods. As a general rule, foods available in health food stores are far more natural than those found elsewhere, but there are exceptions to this. Many valuable food supplements, such as vitamins, minerals, and enzymes, are available in these stores. The average American who has subsisted for years on the typical American diet usually needs many such supplements.

Another feature of the health food store is the type of books and pamphlets that can be obtained there. Literature on almost every known ailment is available. Most of the publications on health problems found in such stores are not available elsewhere. But here again, a word of caution is in order. Some of this literature is nonsense based on pagan philosophy and not on real human experience and nutritional research. Therefore the reader will need to use good common sense and caution in this respect.

There are other aspects of natural health that the patient must observe if he is to really cooperate with God and have the best chance of recovery. He should maintain a positive attitude of optimism and hope. His natural body defenses work best when the emotions are right. He needs to keep as busy as his condition will permit. He needs regular rhythmical exercise, but should avoid strenuous exercise. And by all means he should do all he can to avoid the poisons that are everywhere in our polluted world. For example, auto exhaust fumes contaminate our bodies with many poisons, one of the worst of which is lead. These poisons contribute heavily to the cancer problems. Abundant literature is available giving help on how to reduce our intake of poisons.

One of the saddest scenes that I know of is that of the smoking cancer patient. At a recent cancer symposium, I noticed several patients stubbornly insisting on smoking, even after the master of ceremonies had explained the cancer hazard, the city fire regulations forbidding it, and also the lack of consideration shown to others sitting nearby. The smoking went on. This illustrates a point. Some cancer patients are determined to commit suicide the slow way, and no one is going to deprive them of this privilege. Many cancer patients, like many other persons, have a subconscious death-wish. This of course makes it very difficult on the family and loved ones. If the patient is determined to smoke and fill his lungs with poison, he may as well forget everything in this book. The whole purpose of this book is to encourage the reader to cooperate with God in the prevention and control of cancer. The cancer patient who stubbornly insists on smoking is stubbornly refusing to cooperate with God and he can only expect the worst. "If any man defile the temple of God, him shall God destroy" (1 Cor. 3:17). The patient must make up his mind whether or not he is going to cooperate with God's laws of natural health.

CHOOSE A DIET RICH IN VITAMIN B-17

Even if the dishonest bureaucrats succeed in cutting off all supplies of B-17 tablets and injectables, they can never cut the cancer patient completely off from this wonderful God-given cancer-fighting substance. God knew in advance that Satan would interfere with this marvelous healer, so He placed it abundantly in nature. It is found in over a thousand edible plants in every part of the world. There is no way the bureaucrats can completely stop the flow of B-17 into your body. As the patient continues to study the literature on this subject, he should begin his own lengthy list of foods rich in amygdalin. Of course the availability of these foods will vary with the locality. Here are a few examples:

alfalfa
beans (especially broad beans, Italian beans, lima beans, soy beans)
berries
blackstrap molasses
buckwheat
cassava
flax seed (linseed)
garlic
grasses (especially arrow grass, Johnson grass, sudan grass)
macadamia nuts

millet
oats
peas
rice bran
rye
seeds of fruits of the rose family (apple, apricot, cherry, peach, plum, prune, etc.)
sprouts
vetch.

The distinguishing feature of all foods rich in B-17 is their bitter taste. And unfortunately, Americans have been culturally conditioned to love sweets and to dislike bitter foods. For this reason, nearly all the vitamin B-17 has been removed from the American diet. This is a double tragedy because B-17 fights cancer, and sugar in large quantities encourages cancer.

It is ironical that while a vast and sophisticated machine is attempting to cut off the source of amygdalin, God has placed an abundant supply within easy reach of millions of poor people. Someone asked me what I would do if the FDA succeeds in cutting off all the usual sources of amygdalin, including apricot and peach kernels. I told him that I would go to the abundant Johnson grass fields here in Texas, dig up the tender roots, liquefy them in my blender, and drink me a B-17 cocktail! You see, B-17 is plentiful for those who are willing to seek it. The bureaucrats cannot outwit God!

BECOME FAMILIAR WITH THE MATERIALS OF METABOLIC THERAPY

When we speak of metabolic therapy, we are not speaking of drugs. We are speaking primarily of natural substances that have long been in the human food supply, but which have been refined out of our food in recent decades. Metabolic therapy involves the restoring of these materials to the diet so that the body metabolism can be corrected. In an earlier chapter we spoke briefly concerning the role of vitamins, minerals, enzymes, and proteins in the diet. The cancer patient should spend much time reading the literature that deals with the nutritional role of these and other substances. Of course he will need professional guidance in the field of nutrition, but experience has shown that most patients do not follow professional guidance if they are ignorant of the basic principles of nutrition.

In addition to basic metabolic materials, the cancer patient would be wise to become familiar with the special metabolic substances currently being used by many Laetrile physicians. We will mention a few of these briefly.

Amygdalin, or Vitamin B-17. Much has already been said about this. The reader should remember that the theory is that this substance kills cancer cells by releasing cyanide at the cancer cell, and that it is harmless to other cells. In practice, the results vary from person to person, probably due to the presence or absence of other metabolic substances in the body. Remember that B-17 does not work alone, but is part of a team. B-17 tablets are manufactured in several sizes, the most common being the 500 mg. size. These usually sell from $1.00 to $1.50 each depending on source and quantity purchased. Most physicians I know give from one to six daily, depending on severity of the condition and other factors. Vials of amygdalin in injectable form usually contain three grams and sell for $12.00 to $15.00 each. Most physicians in my acquaintance use from one to six vials weekly. Heavy dosages are often reduced after a few weeks. As the reader can see, B-17 is somewhat expensive, but it still does not compare with modern hospital bills. It is expensive because of bureaucrats' harassment. When the interference is finally stopped, it will probably be manufactured synthetically in vast quantities at reasonable cost.

Pancreatic Enzymes. This is the second most important member of the cancer-fighting team. Just as B-17 is the extrinsic fighter, coming into the body from outside, so likewise the pancreatic enzymes trypsin and chymotrypsin are intrinsic fighters manufactured within the body itself. These enzymes digest food, but they also can digest the protective coating from malignant cells, exposing them to destruction by the white corpuscles. A deficiency of pancreatic enzymes is a major contributing cause of cancer. These digestive enzymes are available in most drug stores and health food stores under a variety of trade names. These tablets may cost from three cents each to 25 cents each, depending on many factors. Some nutritionists recommend up to 20 of the cheaper ones daily, or as many as six or eight of the more expensive ones.

Hydrazine Sulphate. Dr. Dean Burk and several other outstanding scientists are quite excited about the role of this chemical in cancer therapy. This substance helps to protect the liver from being over-worked by the cancer. Malignant cells send out a hormone which goes to the liver and commands the liver to manufacture sugar to feed the cancer. So in effect, the liver is trapped and enslaved by the tumor. This places an enormous load on the liver and can ultimately weaken it. Since the liver is the primary chemical factory of the body, it is the primary cancer-fighting organ and must be protected. Dr. Burk explains that the hydrazine sulphate stops this vicious procedure and releases the liver from this bondage to the cancer. He recommends two 60 mg. capsules daily for the average patient. These are inexpensive and can usually be purchased from the same sources that supply B-17.

Calcium Diorotate. It was formerly thought that after bone tissue was destroyed by cancer, that it could never be rebuilt. Some researchers are now finding that this is not always so. Some recalcification of bone metastases now seems to be possible, and the researchers report that calcium diorotate has been very helpful in this. This is an inexpensive substance.

Pangamic Acid, or Vitamin B-15. This substance has undergone research and development by the same scientists that have done research on B-17. Its primary function is to increase the oxygenation of the blood. In this capacity it has been helpful in the prevention or treatment of cancer, high blood pressure, gangrene, and several other diseases. It is widely used with good success in Russia and West Germany. It is relatively inexpensive.

There are many other metabolic substances that are of benefit to the cancer patient. The reader may study as far as he wishes to go in this field by referring to the reading list.

The reader should realize that this information is given for educational purposes only. Since individual conditions vary, the cancer patient should by all means seek the services of a qualified physician who is skilled in metabolic therapy as well as in general medical practice. The information given here is to enable the patient to cooperate more intelligently with his physician. Help in locating a physician will be given later in this chapter and also in the appendix.

No doubt the reader is wondering where these materials may be purchased. The first place to begin is at your health food store. They will probably have the pancreatic enzymes and possibly some of the other substances. They may also have information on sources of some of the other materials. The appendix at the close of this book will give numerous addresses where materials or information may be obtained.

THE HORMONE TEST FOR EARLY CANCER DETECTION

Cancer can be detected early, long before the physician can locate it by X-ray, and long before the patient feels any symptoms. Unfortunately, the same monopoly that fights natural cancer therapies also fights any simple cancer detection system. The two principal methods in current use to detect cancer are the biopsy and the X-ray. Both of these work only after a tumor is well established and both can spread cancer because they do injury. Once a person has a malignancy located by either of these methods, he has already started down the surgery-radiation-chemotherapy assembly line. If the malignancy is caught early, in its pre-clinical stage, then the patient may never need to get on this assembly line. But our American cancer monopoly doesn't want to lose any prospective customers, so they oppose any simple chemical test that might detect the malignancy early. But opposition or no opposition, the test has been working for many years, and thousands of Americans are learning to protect themselves and their loved ones by this method.

How does it work? Simple! The reader needs to remember that the chemistry of the cancer cell is different from the chemistry of other cells. This makes possible a simple test. Trophoblast cells (and malignant cells, which are the same) produce a hormone known as chorionic gonadotropin. This hormone can be detected in the urine and the amount can be measured, thereby indicating the extent of malignant activity, if any. Of course the test is useless on a pregnant woman because her pregnancy trophoblast cells will always show a positive result.

Some medical laboratories have been forced by court injunction to discontinue giving this test. Why would a judge forbid such a test? No constitutional principle authorizes any court to do such a thing. But when local medical "experts" tell a judge that something is "quackery," he usually believes them. After all, they are the experts, aren't they? Or are they?

I know the test works. I have known of dozens of persons who have sent this test off to distant labs where the patient was completely unknown. Advanced cancer patients always get a high reading. Early cancer patients usually get a medium reading. Healthy persons usually get a low reading. I have known of several persons who detected a malignancy by this method before it showed up in the usual manner. Later it was detected clinically. Instructions and addresses will be given in the appendix.

SEEKING PROFESSIONAL HELP

I realize the dilemma the reader may face at this point, especially if he is a cancer patient. Obviously a matter this serious needs all the professional help one can get. But it is equally obvious that our vast medical-drug-industrial monopoly is trying to make it very difficult for the cancer patient to get the help he needs. Bad as the situation looks, there is still hope. Many cancer patients, perhaps even a majority, can find some measure of professional help in metabolic therapy if they really try. I will give several suggestions. There are numerous organizations dedicated to helping the cancer patient find such help. I will name several in the appendix, but will mention here the one that I believe is most helpful in this respect.

The Committee for Freedom of Choice in Cancer Therapy, a nation-wide organization with headquarters in Los Altos, California, has done a magnificent job of recruiting, educating, and defending such physicians. They maintain a rapidly growing list of highly qualified doctors who have agreed to use metabolic therapy for chronic diseases, including cancer. Most of them will probably include B-17 in the treatment of any patient having a malignant condition. The reader must realize, however, that these physicians will not treat the *cancer*, they will treat the entire health of the patient. But, of course, when the general health of the patient is improved, his body can fight the cancer. In order to contact this organization call telephone number (415) 948-9475. They will supply you with the name of such a physician in your area.

A word of caution: please do not seek an appointment with any of these physicians until the patient is familiar with the legal problems discussed in this book. Great harm is done when an excited patient enters a physician's waiting room and loudly demands that the doctor treat his cancer with Laetrile. This is technically inaccurate and in some states is legally prohibited. But even if the doctor cannot legally treat the cancer with B-17, he can legally treat the patient's health with B-17, and that is even better! As long as the present harassment exists, the patient seeking metabolic treatment for cancer should not mention cancer or B-17 in the physician's waiting room. These can be mentioned later in the quiet privacy of the examining room.

In some cases the nearest such physician may be so far away that the patient chooses not to travel this distance. In such case there are other possibilities. In most large cities there are physicians who use metabolic therapy, including B-17, but they don't let it be known. The most likely prospects are those physicians who describe their field of practice with such terms as *metabolic therapy, nutritional therapy, preventive medicine,* or similar phrases. Your health food store can often recommend a physician who is skilled in this field.

There is one other very definite possibility that will come as a shock to many readers. That is your dentist. Now I realize that there are few dentists, if any, in this country who would openly claim to treat cancer. It would be illegal for them to make such a claim, and it would be professional suicide as well. Nevertheless, many dentists in various parts of the country have "accidentally" brought malignant conditions under control. How? This is not at all surprising if we realize that many dentists are well qualified in the field of metabolic therapy. The dental profession has always placed great emphasis on the role of vitamins, minerals, and other nutritional substances in promoting healthy teeth and gums. There is no doubt that the average dentist in this country is vastly more informed in this field than is the average medical doctor. There is no way that a dentist can correct the body metabolism for oral health without also correcting the body metabolism for over-all health. So many a dentist has accidentally done what he cannot do legally. Sometimes the dentist is as surprised as the patient when there is a distinct improvement in some chronic disease as arthritis, diabetes, or even cancer. There are several large and highly successful metabolic clinics in this country that are staffed by former dentists who "accidentally" discovered the amazing results of a corrected metabolism. At this point we need to repeat a discussion from a former chapter. No doctor can heal you. The body heals itself, under God's direction, if the metabolism is corrected. Therefore, it makes no difference who corrects the metabolism, the results are the same. The metabolic correction may be accomplished under the supervision of a medical doctor, osteopath, chiropractor, naturopath, dentist, or anyone else and the results will be the same. If the patient should be unable to get professional help and was successful in correcting his own metabolism, the results would be the same. Even if a jungle witch doctor should happen to correct the metabolism, the results would be the same. But I don't recommend trying this. I am merely emphasizing that the doctor does not do the healing, the body metabolism does the healing.

We can be grateful to God that the number of courageous doctors who are willing to fight cancer God's way, with metabolic processes, is now on the increase. The appendix will list organizations that help in this respect.

THE READER'S RESPONSIBILITY

Every person who learns this wonderful good news is responsible to share it with others. "Am I my brother's keeper?" Yes! When we see how our wonderful God is bringing cancer and other chronic diseases under control by means of natural substances, we are obligated to share this information with others. But a word of caution, don't go off half-cocked! It may be unwise to bring up this subject until you know what you are talking about. I have often seen a novice in this field become over eager to inform others of these wonderful truths. We must remember that the world hates the gospel and we must use wisdom in presenting it. Likewise this world hates God's way of natural healing. Sometimes the first mention of any natural cancer treatment will bring down an avalanche of opposition and ridicule on the head of the speaker. Does this mean we are to forever remain silent? By no means! But we must get our gun fully loaded before we go into battle. It is best to be thoroughly informed before trying to teach these truths to others. Get the facts and figures. Know what you are talking about and be ready to counter with powerful truth any opposing statement you hear. You will find that the public is in abysmal ignorance concerning this matter. But they have heard the propaganda of the cancer monopoly and they have swallowed it without any investigation. It is difficult to dislodge long-standing prejudices, even when they are totally unfounded.

    One of the most foolish things I know of is for a novice in this field to go ask his doctor if Laetrile is any good. That would be just like a medieval Catholic asking his priest if the Protestant religion was true. In most cases he can expect a dogmatic "no." The reader may feel that his personal physician is the most wonderful and reliable man on earth. But please remember that he probably is not a B-17 researcher and he doesn't know anything about it except the propaganda he has read. If he receives the AMA-FDA propaganda, then he will believe B-17 is useless. Even good men are inclined to follow such prejudice without knowing the facts. So in most cases the family doctor is not the place to get correct B-17 information. A far better course of action is for the reader to *tell* his doctor, not *ask* him! But before you tell him, first learn what you are talking about. After you have read several books and have seen several patients improve on B-17, you will know vastly more about it than your doctor does. Then you can tell him forcefully and with conviction. You can counter his hearsay with your known facts. You may be fortunate enough to start your physician on the right track and indirectly save many lives. It can be done. I have seen a persistent little lady with limited formal education but plenty of facts finally convince a brilliant physician about the reality of B-17.

There are others besides the medical profession who should feel the pressure of an informed public. Those who learn about B-17 should take advantage of every opportunity to get the facts before congressmen and other public officials and to contact the newspapers and other media whenever possible. Every person who knows the truth about the B-17 controversy should spread the good word wherever possible. But again, be thoroughly convinced yourself before you attempt to convince others.

The Responsibility of Christian Leaders. It is sincerely hoped that these lines come to the attention of many preachers of the gospel and other Christian workers. Brethren, I know full well that the average preacher already has more responsibilities than he can carry. I also know that Christian leaders must put spiritual matters first and must sometimes resist the pressures of other matters that seem secondary. But brethren, we do have a responsibility under God to try and rescue some of the millions that are dying needlessly in our great cancer slaughter. If it had been in your power to stop Hitler's slaughter of twelve million innocent civilians, would you have declined on the ground that you had to stick with spiritual duties? Well, at the rate we are going, the cancer slaughter just in our country alone will outdo Hitler within thirty years! Can we stand aloof from the controversy and refuse to get involved? The Word of God has already spoken very clearly on this question:

> If thou forbear to deliver them that are drawn unto death, and those that are ready to be

slain; If thou sayest, Behold, we knew it not; doth not he that pondereth the heart consider it? and he that keepeth thy soul, doth not he know it? and shall not he render to every man according to his works?   (Prov. 24: 11-12)

Could anything be more plain? The Christian who learns the truth about our national cancer disgrace has a responsibility to the poor victims who are "drawn unto death" and "ready to be slain." The child of God who knows about the benefits of God-given B-17 cannot be silent. It will do no good for us to plead ignorance. We could know the truth if we would put out some effort! "If thou sayest, behold we knew it not; doth not He that pondereth the heart consider it?" According to this plain statement from the Word of God, many Christian leaders are going to have to give account for the careless neglect of multitudes who were needlessly dying. Ignorance is no excuse! The facts are available. We can know if we will!

Remember the story of the good Samaritan? Why did the priest and the Levite pass by the dying man? Because they were busy with what they considered spiritual business!

One of the most terrible aspects of our national cancer disgrace is the awful plight of the terminal cancer patient. The Food and Drug Administration will not give him permission to get pain relief with harmless vitamin B-17. So the physician gives him massive doses of morphine to relieve his agony. During the last weeks of his life he is no longer a human being. He is a narcotic addict. He is a mere vegetable! Under the powerful influence of these deadly narcotics, his entire personality can change. Men who have been saintly Christians for many years can revert back to long-forgotten evil ways. Cursing, obscene language, and blasphemous words can come from the lips of one who has for years worshipped and praised God. Of course he is not responsible because this is not the expression of his true personality. It is merely the resurgence of his old natural life which has long been held in check by his new Christian nature. But nevertheless, what a terrible shock for the loved ones! How cruel to reduce a man of God to such shame just before his death! What a victory for the devil! And we ministers stand idly by and let this happen! It is our duty to inform such families of the pain-relieving properties of B-17. Most terminal patients find that with vitamin B-17 they need little or no narcotics. Every terminal cancer patient should have the right to die with dignity, with all of his senses intact, and with a minimum of pain. Our present cancer monopoly would even deny him that.

Another important point for the preacher of the gospel: how many times have we gone to the hospital to tell the dying cancer patient about salvation through Christ, only to find him so stupefied with drugs that he could not understand! Can you think of anything more terrible?

Not only is our cancer monopoly responsible for his death, they are also responsible for his eternally lost soul! This needless tragedy can often be prevented by a simple, God-given vitamin. Preacher, don't you think it is our duty to try and prevent this? We can inform others of the existence of vitamin B-17. We may not feel it wise to insist on its use, but we can at least reveal its existence and let the family make the decision on its use.

The Responsibility of Christians in the Healing Professions. The Christian physician who learns the truth about metabolic therapy will face a dilemma indeed. If he follows the truth in this field, he runs the risk of losing his license, losing his hospital privileges, or even possible arrest. At the very least he will suffer ridicule and ostracism from his peers. At first this will seem like too great a price to pay. But wait a minute! What is a Christian anyway? A Christian is one who has come to realize that this present world system is evil (Gal. 1:4) and that Satan is the god of this world (2 Cor. 4:4). He has repented of his sins, he has trusted in the sacrifice of Jesus Christ to pay for those sins, and he has yielded himself to the risen Lord. This automatically means that he has turned his back on this God-hating world. One of the basic principles of Christianity is that the believer is to be separated from the world (2 Cor. 6:17). He is not to be controlled any longer by the world's principles of greed and fame (1 John 2:15-17).

Another basic principle of the Christian life is that we are to be motivated by loving concern for others, not by our own selfish desires. In fact, our dedication to Christ and to others is to be so firm that we will lay down our lives before we will rebel against our living Lord. None of us would be Christians today, none of us would have even heard the gospel, if the martyrs of former days had not died to bring us the gospel. All the liberties we cherish so dearly were won for us by those who were willing to lay down their lives for the truth. Whether it be in the field of religion, or government, or medical science, truth as been won by those courageous men who held truth more dear than life itself. Are those days gone forever? Are there no more men who will lay down their lives for the truth of God? Have we now become a nation of spineless cowards? Every informed Christian doctor, every Christian nurse, every child of God in the healing professions who learns the truth about metabolic therapy faces a most serious responsibility. What will your choice be? Will you protect your own comfortable income and your own professional prestige and let people die needlessly? What will you say when you stand before the Lord Jesus Christ? May God have mercy on us puny, spineless creatures if we keep silent in the day of slaughter. Thank God there are many believers in the healing professions who put God and others and truth ahead of personal gain. They are standing up. They are helping the poor cancer victims at risk to themselves. They are crying out for the truth and are winning others over to their point of view. They are showing that they are made of the same material as Vesaleus and Harvey and Semmelweis. May their tribe rapidly increase!

The Responsibility of Christians in Government Agencies. I cannot think of a more miserable person on the face of the globe than a child of God who finds himself to be a helpless pawn of those cruel agencies of government that suppress nutritional therapy. How terrible it will be to arrest some godly doctor for treating diseases with the substances God has always used to treat diseases, and then finally to stand before the God that made the healing substances. How embarrassing! It is my firm belief that any Christian who knows the Word of God will realize (once he gets the facts) that Satan is behind all persecution of natural healing.

No doubt these lines will be read by such government agents. I sincerely hope so. I would like nothing better than to help these unhappy persons to escape from their terrible predicament. How about it, Mr. FDA agent, are you a born-again child of God or not? Have you been saved from your sins by repenting of those sins and trusting in the Lord Jesus Christ? If not, then you have far more serious troubles facing you. God's Word says you will face the vengeance of eternal fire (2 Thess. 1:8-9) just like any other sinner if you do not get saved. On the other hand, Mr. Government Agent, if you are a born-again child of God, you still have a problem. Are you going to help persecute God's men for using God's materials to help God's people? You do indeed have a problem! You had better use all the influence you have to persuade your agency to discontinue this unconstitutional harassment. If you do not, then someday the Lord will ask you why!

Don't forget that government agents get cancer too. And there is an often repeated principle in the Bible that states that he who sets a trap will fall therein (Prov. 26:27). Now what is likely to happen to you if you cooperate with this terrible trap that is destroying so many helpless cancer victims? God may just let you get caught in that trap! You had better work for the full legalization of vitamin B-17 and all other nutritional therapies. Some day you or a dear loved one may desperately need those very therapies. Think it over!

Some physicians have been cruelly persecuted by government agencies for using Laetrile. Yet in some cases the FDA agents, the judges, and the prosecuting attorneys have later contracted cancer and have gone to these same physicians for help. You see, persecutors do get cancer themselves! And not all will be fortunate enough to find one of these kind Laetrile physicians. Many who war against God's cancer control will die of agonizing cancer themselves.

There *is* something we can do about cancer.

God has provided some help, and we can cooperate with Him no matter how great the opposition. We can do much for ourselves, and we can do much to help other cancer victims. I am so grateful to God that I learned this, even though I had to become a cancer victim myself in order to discover it.

"In every thing give thanks"
(1 Thessalonians 5:18)

I can thank God for cancer, because it impressed upon me this basic Bible principle—

PRINCIPLE NO. 11
WE ARE ALL TERMINAL!

This is the most encouraging chapter in this entire book. Don't let the title fool you into thinking that this is a morbid discussion. By no means! This chapter is designed to relieve fear, to give hope and encouragement, and to help the patient face the future with understanding, with confidence, and to be fully prepared for whatever may come.

THERE IS NOTHING UNUSUAL ABOUT BEING TERMINAL

When a patient is informed by his physician that the disease is incurable and that the end is near, he is overwhelmed by many emotions. Of course there is dread of death, the fear of the unknown, the shock, the helplessness, perhaps even panic and anger. But among the many negative emotions there is also the feeling of loneliness, the sense of being somehow separated from the rest of society, in a class by himself. And this is indeed depressing. We all want to belong, to be accepted as a normal member of the group. But now we are not so sure that we are accepted. Now we are strange. We wonder if perhaps others are looking at us as some kind of freak, perhaps as unwanted, perhaps even as "unclean." We are not quite sure how we fit into society now.

In response to this, I could say many things. First, dear terminal patient, please realize that you are perfectly normal and that everybody else is in the same boat you are in. You see, *we are all terminal!* When God placed Adam in the garden and warned him not to eat of the forbidden fruit, He said, "In the day that thou eatest thereof thou shalt surely die" (Gen. 2:17). When Adam rebelled against his Creator, the sentence of death fell upon him and the process of death began to work in his body and in his entire being. We have all descended from Adam and we have all inherited this death sentence from him (Rom. 5:12). So you see, we are all dying. The baby starts dying as soon as he is born. Death is gnawing away at all of us all the time. So there is really nothing unusual about us when the doctor tells us we are going to die. What is so odd about that? We have been in the process of dying for years! We are all alike in this respect. The only difference is that some of us are nearer than others.

The terminal cancer patient may still be discouraged because it appears that he will not live as long as others. I wouldn't be too sure about that. God's Word warns us that life is very uncertain for all of us, not just for cancer victims (James 4:14). I knew of a "terminal" cancer patient that enjoyed a measure of normal living for thirteen years. I also knew of a young physician in the very prime of life who died suddenly in a traffic accident. You see, we are all terminal, and we really don't know who is going to terminate first. So, cancer patient, by all means don't feel strange or embarrassed, you are no more terminal than anybody else!

THE TERMINAL PATIENT HAS CERTAIN ADVANTAGES

Do you mean there is something good about being told that I only have so many months to live? Absolutely! The doctor's estimate is often wrong (especially if the patient is using B-17), but it is often fairly accurate. This has some definite advantages. First, it helps us to realize the certainty of death. Of course, everyone knows he is going to die, or at least he says he knows it. But does he *really* know it? Apparently not. Sometimes it takes quite a shock to make us realize that death is real. If it takes a terminal malignant condition to make us face the reality of death, then that is fine! It is far better than plunging headlong into a sudden death that we never really believed was coming. The second advantage is that we have a better idea of the time of our departure and can therefore make better preparations. Who would want to make a long trip without having any idea at all when his plane was leaving?

This book was written primarily for Christians. Assuming that the reader is a terminal patient and also a true believer in Jesus Christ, then you have been chosen by our Lord for a special service. You are in a position to show others that God is able to sustain you in the face of death. The young healthy Christian can *say* that the grace of God is sufficient in such an hour, but he cannot demonstrate it. So you have an advantage. You can demonstrate how the grace of God works in this particular situation. Don't miss this opportunity!

The person who is near the end of this life is often a more effective witness for Christ than he formerly was. It is so easy for the world to shake off the testimony of the average Christian. But the words of a dying person have a special power. People often listen to such words with great interest. So use those words to point others to Jesus Christ who died to pay for our sins. Christ Himself stopped dying long enough to save a poor lost sinner. Perhaps you can stop dying long enough to point another to the Lamb of God.

Terminal patient, you are to be envied. If you die sooner than the rest of us, that just means you will see Jesus before we do. There's nothing bad about that! That is the true goal of every human soul. Don't shrink from it!

IF YOU ARE NOT SAVED

Possibly these lines will be read by one who does not have this joyous hope in Christ because you have never been saved. Then if your malignant condition leads you to find salvation in Christ, you can thank God for your malignancy.

It is possible for you to know for sure that you have eternal life; God wants you to know.

> These things have I written unto you that believe on the name of the Son of God; that ye may know that ye have eternal life, and that ye may believe on the name of the Son of God. (1 John 5:13)

In order to know that you have eternal life, there are a few Bible truths you must understand. First, you must understand that you are a sinner.

> As it is written, There is none righteous, no, not one. (Rom. 3:10) For all have sinned, and come short of the glory of God. (Rom. 3:23)

Next, you must understand that because of our

sin we deserve death, both physical death and eternal death.

> For the wages of sin is death; but the gift of God is eternal life through Jesus Christ our Lord. (Rom. 6:23)

Next, you must understand that Jesus Christ the Son of God has already died to pay for your sins.

> But God commendeth his love toward us, in that, while we were yet sinners, Christ died for us. (Rom. 5:8)

Finally, you must believe on the resurrected Christ, trust in Him, accept Him as your Saviour from sin.

> For whosoever shall call upon the name of the Lord shall be saved. (Rom. 10:13)

Have you trusted Him? Now rest your case completely in His hands. Be assured that He will never leave you or forsake you (Hebrews 13:5). Death for the believer will be a great step forward, a great victory. Death is just the shedding of the present handicaps and the entrance into the full sonship of God. Death for the believer is a triumphant success.

If you have just trusted Christ, then you are a new baby in the family of God (John 3:3, 1 John 5:1). Christian babies grow on the Word of God (1 Pet. 2:2-3). Let the remaining days of your life be spent in growing stronger as a Christian.

Read the gospel of John for strength and encouragement, then the remainder of the New Testament. Find a church that really preaches the Bible and tries to win people to Christ. If physically able to do so, be baptized to show what Christ has done for you, and attend every service of the church you possibly can. Not only will you receive strength and encouragement, you may be surprised at how God will use you to be a blessing to someone else!

YOU MAY NEVER SEE DEATH

We so often speak of the absolute certainty of death, but there is no such absolute certainty. If the reader has not been familiar with this Biblical teaching, it may seem strange at first, but it is a fact. Multitudes of human beings will never die, and if you are a born-again child of God, you may be one of them. We have these wonderful promises from the Word of God:

> For the Lord Himself shall descend from heaven with a shout, with the voice of the archangel, and with the trump of God: and the dead in Christ shall rise first: Then we which are alive and remain shall be caught up together with them in the clouds, to meet the Lord in the air: and so shall we ever be with the Lord. (1 Thess. 4:16-17)

> Behold, I shew you a mystery; We shall not all sleep, but we shall all be changed, In a

moment, in the twinkling of an eye, at the last trump: for the trumpet shall sound, and the dead shall be raised incorruptible, and we shall be changed. (1 Cor. 15:51-52)

O death, where is thy sting? O grave, where is thy victory? (1 Cor. 15:55)

But thanks be to God, which giveth us the victory through our Lord Jesus Christ. (1 Cor. 15:57)

There is good reason to believe that many Christians living today will be in this group that escapes death. Bible prophecy even now seems to be in the process of fulfillment. The coming of our Lord Jesus Christ is drawing nearer. Wouldn't it be wonderful to be ushered into His presence without dying? When we see Jesus, we will be made like Him, and that means perfect in body and in soul and spirit. No more sin, no more human weakness, and no more disease (1 John 3:2).

Christian friend, even if Christ does not return in time to prevent your death, you are still going to get a new and perfect body at the time of His return. This is a clear promise from the Word of God.

For our conversation [citizenship] is in heaven, from whence also we look for the Saviour, the Lord Jesus Christ: Who shall change our vile body, that it may be fashioned like unto His glorious body, according to the working whereby he is able even to subdue all things unto himself. (Phil. 3:20-21)

If you depart from this life, it will merely mean that you are moving out of the house that is no longer fit for habitation (2 Cor. 5:1-4). You will go immediately into the glorious presence of Christ in Heaven (2 Cor. 5:8; Phil. 1:23). You will never go into the grave at all. The thing that will be placed in the casket is definitely not you; it is merely a vacant house. You yourself will be with Christ. This means your personality, your consciousness, the real you. But you will not remain forever in spirit form. When Jesus returns, your old body will be raised and transformed into a new and perfect body. Your spirit will return into this new glorified Christlike body, and you will rejoice with Him forever. So rejoice now, and look forward to the good things that lie ahead. You were created in the beginning for a purpose. That purpose is to love Christ, to have fellowship with Him, and to bring honor to Him. If you are saved, then that purpose has been accomplished to a certain extent. You can thank God that it is going to be accomplished perfectly. Life has finally found meaning and purpose. It is vastly better to be a terminal cancer victim in fellowship with Christ than to be in the prime of health and lost outside of His will. Don't you think so?

IF I SHOULD DIE OF CANCER

For seven years I have kept a serious malignancy under control by means of vitamin B-17 and other natural metabolic substances. But I know that I am not going to live forever in this present frail body. If Jesus doesn't come in the next few years, then I too, like millions before me, will enter into the presence of Christ by the avenue of death. This fact does not terrify me one bit. I am quite sure that the Christ who has been so gracious to me all the days of my life, will be sufficient in the hour of death. He has already passed through the experience of death and has conquered it for us. The sting of death is gone for the believer.

If I die of cancer, I expect some may rejoice over this. Since I have aligned myself so definitely on the side of God-given B-17, it may be that some of the enemies of B-17 class me as their enemy also. Let me make it clear that I am no man's enemy, even if he should class me as his enemy.

In case some government agent or some servant of organized medicine, dedicated to the destruction of the Laetrile traffic, should read these lines, let me say a word to you. If I should die of cancer, you need not rejoice. I am with the Lord Jesus Christ and you aren't. I am a million times better off than you and I wouldn't consider for one moment trading places with you.

In case I should die of cancer, some may use

this as proof that B-17 is worthless. This would be the height of stupidity! Mr. FDA Agent, if I die of cancer, it is not the fault of B-17, but it is to some extent *your fault!* For the first 53 years of my life I ate the typical American junk diet, the garbage you approve of, with all the nourishment refined out and all the poisons put in, *with your permission.* I received the disgracefully low vitamin levels you recommended. I ate the poisonous white bread with dozens of God-given nutrients taken out and with a few minute nutrients put in, which you called *enriched bread!* So don't blame B-17, blame the disgraceful American diet that you defended so many years! And for what reason? What large industry were you protecting?

Mr. FDA, there is another reason why I might have lived longer if it had not been for your interference. Your opposition to B-17 was wrong, criminally wrong in the sight of God. It cannot be justified on any grounds. The fact that you considered it worthless is no excuse. You know full well that you allowed hundreds of worthless substances to be used, along with dozens of definitely harmful substances. So your opposition to B-17 is totally without excuse. This opposition was only to protect the economic interests of some other group. But your harassment did serve one purpose. It made B-17 difficult to obtain and drove up the price until most of us could not afford it. What did you do with all that B-17 you seized? Do you realize that thousands were dying in pain while you stole their relief and kept it locked up in some warehouse? Or did you sell it on the black market? What will you say when you stand before God? What excuse can you give that will satisfy Him? No, don't say that my death proves B-17 worthless. Say instead that B-17 kept me going for many years but that you were able to reduce my supply and shorten my life. But don't rejoice over your "victory." I wouldn't trade places with you.

How about it, Mr. Agent? Have you been saved from your sins? You need Jesus Christ just like the rest of us. No matter how many innocent cancer victims you have killed, Christ will still save you. Trust Him today, and start serving on His side. He has a purpose for your life. If you will yield to Him, He will use you. Among other things, He will use you to defend His natural treatments of disease, just as in the past you have fought against His therapies. And in that kind of service you will find that you bring honor to God, blessings to your fellow man, and a sense of fulfillment to yourself.

It is my sincere desire that all who read this book will come to a saving knowledge of the Lord Jesus Christ, and will find joy and satisfaction in His service. The purpose of this book has been to honor Christ and benefit men. If the reader feels that it contains errors, then I beg your indulgence for those errors. I tried sincerely to get the facts straight. If some statements seem a bit harsh, then again I beg your indulgence. Harshness is not my nature. But when millions are dying and are denied a God-given relief, someone needs to cry aloud. If even one life is saved because of any strong words I may have used, you will excuse them, won't you?

And so we are all terminal. I have known this for many years. We are all dying, eternity-bound souls. But since I have been a cancer patient, I have realized this more fully. This present world has become less important, and eternal life with Christ has become more real. Since it took cancer to bring me to this deeper realization, I can say, "Thank God I have cancer." My cancer led me to write this book. I trust some will be helped by it. Perhaps you too can thank God that I had cancer.

> And we know that all things work together for good to them that love God, to them who are the called according to his purpose. (Rom. 8:28)

"In every thing give thanks"
(1 Thessalonians 5:18)

I can thank God even for cancer,
because it led me to see clearly
this serious Christian responsibility—

PRINCIPLE NO. 12: HONEST MEN MUST SUPPORT FREEDOM OF CHOICE

One of the most significant movements in America today is the movement to allow physicians and patients Freedom of Choice in Cancer Therapy. For decades the American Cancer Monopoly has decreed that surgery, radiation and chemotherapy must be used even if they don't work and even if physician and patient do not want these therapies. The Monopoly has also decreed that natural, God-given, non-toxic treatments must not be used, even if they are highly successful and both patient and doctor wish to use them. I challenge anyone to find a more vicious example of tyranny in all the annals of human history! Likewise, the movement for freedom of choice in this area, when successful, will prove to be one of the greatest victories for human rights the world has ever seen.

WHO SUPPORTS FREEDOM OF CHOICE?

There are at least three groups of people who are vitally interested in the success of this movement, each for different reasons.

Health. Many are interested for reasons of health and physical welfare. They have long been aware that natural avenues of health have been superior to the un-natural route of man-made chemicals. To them, this battle for freedom of choice in cancer therapy is one more chapter in a centuries-old fight for the right to cooperate with nature in maintaining a healthy body.

Freedom. Others are interested for reasons of political freedom. They may not understand the value of vitamin B-17, but they see the senseless, bureaucratic opposition to this vitamin as another example of creeping collectivism. These defenders of our freedom are acutely aware that ever-expanding government is seeking to control every detail of our lives. They want freedom of choice in cancer therapy because they want FREEDOM! And this is wise. A person does not have to understand the value of B-17 in order to support it. He only has to be aware of the growing trend toward oppression and tyranny. When Americans lose the right to care for their own bodies with natural food extracts, then our freedoms are gone.

Christianity. There is yet a third group that is concerned about the movement for freedom of choice. They are informed, Bible-believing Christians. This is not to imply that all such believers are in the group, but merely that the group consists of such believers. This group is concerned for freedom of choice for several reasons. They believe that God has provided for healing in nature, and this belief is based on experience and also on Biblical suggestions. These Christians are also aware, from Bible prophecies, that Satan is seeking to set up a one-world government of absolute tyranny. They see the senseless opposition to God's healing remedies as a part of the trend toward the tyrannical world-government of the anti-Christ.

From these facts it is clear that every honest American, Christian or otherwise, can find at least one reason why he cannot, in good conscience, refuse to cooperate with the movement for freedom of choice. Surely we are for God, rather than anti-god! Surely we are in favor of that which is natural more than that which is against nature! Surely we are for human liberty and not human oppression! Every honest citizen who will search his own heart will find one or more reasons why he must support freedom of choice. The only reasons for opposing freedom of choice are economics, pride, and power.

THE CHRISTIAN'S RESPONSIBILITY TO HEAL

Many Christians and some Christian leaders are opposed to any involvement in the problems of public health. Some contend that "we are only interested in the souls of men." This suggests that we are our brother's keeper in relation to his soul but not in relation to his physical life or death. In many cases we will have no opportunity to deal with a man's soul unless we can keep him alive a little longer. Such an attitude reveals an appalling ignorance of the basic principles of the Christian faith. The word of God clearly states that the Lord is concerned for our "spirit and soul and body" (1 Thess. 5:23). Jesus instructed His disciples to "heal the sick" among other things. Then later in His final Great Commission to His followers, He instructed them to teach others to "observe all things whatsoever I have commanded you" (Matt. 28:19-20). Clearly then, believers in all periods of time are commanded to heal the sick as well as to evangelize the unbelievers. To use evangelism as an excuse to ignore healing is to rebel against the plain words of our Lord Jesus Christ.

Since we have this Christian obligation to heal, what methods shall we use? A little common sense will give the answer. We may occasionally choose to use man-made methods of healing, but only if they do not conflict with God's natural healing methods. For example, as Christians we are not wise to use the powerful, man-made, chemical poisons that destroy God's natural immunilogical system. This rules out a large portion of currently used radiation and chemotherapy. While we may cautiously employ some of the man-made therapies, the Christian philosophy of healing will compel us to emphasize natural, God-given methods.

Let me summarize. Jesus commanded His followers to heal. Surely He meant for us to use the methods He placed in nature as Creator. These natural methods basically involve nutrition, but as a science are sometimes known as metabolic therapy. Therefore every Christian is morally obligated to understand metabolic therapy, to support it, to encourage others to use it, and to defend those courageous doctors and others who are being persecuted for promoting natural healing. Since metabolic therapy merely means cooperating with God's design in nature, we must see that the current persecution of this therapy is part of the program of anti-God.

WHICH SIDE ARE YOU ON?

LEVELS OF LEGAL AUTHORITY

The Christian who wishes to stand up for nutritional therapy is often hampered by confusion over the legal status of these therapies. Since power-hungry bureaucrats want to suppress these God-given therapies, they attempt to use the law as a tool of suppression. Christians then draw back and refuse to cooperate with God for fear they may be doing something "illegal." This confusion results in a defeat for God and a victory for the forces of anti-god. To correct this confusion, every Christian needs to have a clear understanding of the various levels of legal authority. Not everything that is said to be "legal" or "illegal" rests on equal footing, for some law is higher than other law.

We can grade the levels of legal authority something like this, starting with the highest level and progressing downward to the lower levels of authority. (1) The law of God. (2) The constitution of the United States. (3) Statutes enacted by Congress or State Legislature. (4) Court interpretations based on these statutes. (5) Clearly written bureaucratic guidelines based on specific statutes. (6) Bureaucratic procedures having no written basis.

What should be the Christian attitude toward these various levels of legal authority? While we may feel that we must obey them all, there is no Christian principle that compels us to respect them all. In fact, it is often impossible to respect them all. For example, bureaucratic procedures often flagrantly violate the constitution. If I then respect such a bureaucratic procedure, I am showing disrespect for the constitution. In order to honor the higher law, I am compelled to oppose the lower law. Therefore the Christian who humbly submits without question to every action of every government agency proves himself to be ignorant of our legal structure and also too cowardly to stand up for the highest levels of legal authority.

Let me cite a recent example. For over a century, vitamin B-17 and other natural food substances have been used and shipped freely without any governmental regulations, just like fruit juices or any other food extracts. Only recently, when these substances were found to be helpful in cancer prevention, did government bureaucrats step in to prevent their shipment into this country. Dying cancer patients who have been abandoned by "orthodox" medicine attempt to import B-17 (apricot extract) into this country. The B-17 is seized at the border. When the border officials are questioned as to what legal document gives them authority to seize this material, they can give no answer. Notice this horrible state of affairs! They admit that there is no statute forbidding the shipment of this substance. Vitamin B-17 does not even appear on any FDA list of forbidden materials. Clearly then, the seizure of B-17 is based on level (6) of legal authority as listed above, a bureaucratic procedure having no formal written basis. This action not only condemns cancer patients to needless suffering and early death, but it also violates the highest of all laws, (1) the law of God, and (2) the Constitution of the United States. Fortunately, a United States District Court and a United States Court of Appeals have recently recognized these facts and have accordingly ruled in favor of the cancer patients. Unfortunately, the process of restoring constitutional freedoms is very slow and it will be some time before the bureaucratic harrassment of cancer patients is stopped completely and on a nationwide scale.

Christians need to understand that our constitution provided for only three branches of government: executive, legislative, and judicial. But we have developed a powerful bureaucracy that is in fact a fourth branch of government. And in practice we are ruled by this fourth branch of unelected rulers, while the three constitutional branches have abandoned much of their authority to the bureaucrats.

The Christian then who blindly supports every bureaucratic action because he wants to be "legal" may in fact be supporting an illegal action and may be tearing down the highest levels of legal authority. God will hold us responsible to support that which is really law. We will not be excused if we take the easy route and support bureaucratic procedures that merely appear on the surface to be law. Christians must remember that Satan is a deceiver. It is to his advantage to make non-law appear to be law, and thus to confuse honest men.

DO YOU HAVE THE COURAGE TO STAND UP FOR THE CONSTITUTION AND THE HIGHER LAW?

WHEN LAW IS USED TO PERVERT JUSTICE

Law is an instrument for administering justice. Because it is an imperfect instrument, it often fails to accomplish its purpose. Justice is an eternal and unchanging principle, because it is based on the nature of God, His decrees, and the nature of man. Justice is fundamental and unchanging while law is often fickle and changing. God demands that men must be just in their dealings with other men, but He does not require that the laws be written in any special form. He will accept no excuse for injustice, whether it be "legal" injustice or illegal injustice.

In theory, laws are enacted to promote fairness and justice in human relationships. But in practice, such is often not the case. God's word makes it clear that men are capable of monstrous evil, and that a favorite tool of evil men is to pervert law toward their own selfish ends. So law, instead of being an instrument of justice, becomes instead an instrument of injustice, oppression, and cruelty.

> "Therefore the law is slacked, and judgment doth never go forth: for the wicked doth compass about the righteous; therefore wrong judgment proceedeth" (Habakkuk 1:4).

It has been a fact of history that good men are concerned with justice, while evil men care not for justice but are only interested in manipulating the technicalities of the law. Why? Because pure justice can never be selfish, while law can easily be used to promote selfish ends. One Supreme Court justice long ago stated that law without justice is tyranny. How true!

The prophets of God in the Old Testament were harrassed and some were even executed by a perverted application of "law." John the Baptist stood up against the illegal practices of local rulers, demanded that they obey the law, and lost his head for it. Jesus was crucified by the methods of law, but in violation of clearly written principles of law. The Apostle Paul was imprisoned illegally by the Roman authorities, and while still in prison was able to put fear into the hearts of those authorities by exposing their illegal practice (Acts 16:35-38). That is the kind of Christian courage that is needed today. Thousands were burned at the stake during the Inquisition for believing in Christ, all by apparently legal procedures. Hitler butchered twelve million innocent persons, and many conscientious Germans cringed at this, but then eased their conscience by saying it was the law. History is filled with such examples of law being used to pervert justice.

The thoughtful Christian knows that such action will not stand the test of divine judgment. God is not interested in legal technicalities, but rather in honesty, righteousness, and justice. In fact, those who pervert law to accomplish injustice are under the most severe anathema of God, because their actions are based on wicked hypocrisy and result in severe cruelty.

Let us look at a more modern example. In a recent California court case, a dying cancer victim asked the court for permission to purchase vitamin B-17 to relieve his suffering. He had been given up by the medical establishment; they said they could do nothing more for him. All parties in the case recognized that the B-17 was harmless, yet the court ruled that he could not have this God-given relief. He died in misery, and some of the government agents were delighted at their victory. Such "legal" torture and manslaughter continues the age-old practices of Hitler and the Spanish Inquisition. Every decent American must shudder in horror at shame at such examples of human injustice and cruelty. I tremble to think what will happen to such persecutors when the Supreme Court of Heaven meets! We will then see clearly that the action that passed as "legal" was in fact grossly illegal. God will punish injustice, and injustice under the guise of "legality," far from being excused will receive the greater damnation for its hypocrisy.

WHICH SIDE WILL YOU BE ON IN THAT DAY?

WE ARE RESPONSIBLE TO CHANGE UNJUST AND ILLEGAL LAWS

To submit quietly to unjust laws and then to defend our inaction on the grounds of "good citizenship" is hypocritical in the extreme. Such neglect of duty is contrary to Christian principles and is inconsistent with the principles of freedom that underlie our nation. All that is necessary for the triumph of evil is that good men do nothing. Our failure to resist unjust laws cannot truly be called Christian, for it is in fact anti-Christian. Sometimes our lazy, irresponsible submission to the shell of "legality" is nothing but an excuse for the shirking of our responsibility.

Let me cite the example of Nehemiah in the Old Testament. Cyrus the supreme Emporer had issued an imperial decree authorizing the Jews to rebuild the city of Jerusalem. Furthermore he had decreed that all local authorities give assistance to the Jews in this project. Soon after the work started, local bureaucrats ordered it stopped. Most of God's people sheepishly submitted to this "law," which was actually nothing but an illegal bureaucratic decree. No doubt some of them boasted of their good, law-abiding citizenship because they had submitted to this bureaucratic edict. But in fact they were cooperating with a crime because the law of the empire had authorized this project and the law of God had required it. So these lazy Jews submitted to a lower law and violated the higher laws. Their pious submission to "law" was merely a hypocritical excuse for their failure to perform their duty, and God had to raise up special prophets to stir the people to action (Haggai 1:2-4).

But Nehemiah the man of God was not one of these lazy ones. With holy indignation he denounced the greedy bureaucrats for their lawlessness. He stirred the people out of their lethargy. He demanded a legal appeal to the highest court of the land. And when the emperial records were searched, he was vindicated. The rebuilding of the wall was ruled legal, and the bureaucratic opposition was ruled illegal. And the work of God went forward. Thank God for men of courage like Nehemiah! In order to stand up for higher law, he went through a period in which he seemed to be a lawbreaker. No doubt some of his pious but ignorant countrymen criticized him for not submitting to bureaucratic law!

This teaches us a vastly significant truth. Christians must be willing to stand up for justice even if we pay for it without lives. Surely then we must be willing to be misunderstood and even be called a "lawbreaker" if this is the price we must pay to defend justice and higher law.

At no place in this book do I advocate rebellion against true law. But often a lower law contradicts a higher law, and we are trapped in a position where it is impossible to support both. Because of our complex legal structure, there are times when an illegal law cannot be changed unless someone is willing to test it by breaking it. Often the courts have refused to rule on the constitutionality of a statute until someone violates it. This places us in the uncomfortable position where the only way to get rid of an illegal law is to violate it so it can be tested in the courts. No sensible person can class this type of action as un-Christian or un-American. While God's Word does command us to obey law, the context makes it clear that the laws referred to are laws against violence. When a petty bureaucratic edict has no relation to crime or violence or morality, when it is contrary to the constitution, when it cannot be tested in court until someone violates it, then such a legal test cannot rightly be classed as "lawbreaking". And such action, far from being un-Christian, may in fact be motivated by the highest of Christian principles. Remember that God is not primarily concerned with our technicalities; He tests everything by the motives of the heart. Incidentally, the idea I have just outlined is not new The Federal courts long ago ruled that no one should obey an unconstitutional law.

Some Christians may find it difficult to accept this idea that it is sometimes righteous to violate a bad law in order to get rid of it. I can give an example that anyone can understand. In the past, certain cities and states enacted laws forbidding black people to drink at public fountains. We now know these laws were unconstitutional and wrong. But how could such an illegal law be changed? The constitution does not automatically correct bad laws. They must be violated in order to be tested. So it seemed that the only way to change this law was to break it. The black man who tested this law by drinking from the white man's fountain was jailed as a criminal. Some of his thoughtless Christian friends may have rebuked him as a "lawbreaker." But when his case was tested in court, it was ruled that his action was legal and that those who arrested him were illegal. Do we now say that this black man was a lawbreaker? Certainly not! We now realize that he was defending the highest principle of law. Higher courts have consistently indicated that this is the proper course of action to take in case of an unconstitutional law. How stupid we are then to class such persons as "lawbreakers." Sometimes a person must sacrifice himself to an unjust law in order to remove it.

Why don't we learn our lesson? When an honest and courageous man violates a petty bureaucratic decree, when no principle of violence or morals is involved, when no one is harmed, when there is no selfish motive, when his only purpose is to test the constitutionality of the decree, how dare we brand him as a criminal! To do so merely exposes our own total lack of justice and our ignorance of the lessons of history! History will teach us that such courageous persons have been heroes, patriots, and pioneers for freedom and right. And conversely, those who defend unjust and unconstitutional laws under the guise of being "legal" are themselves both cowards and lawbreakers.

Let me cite some more recent examples. A few years ago the California Health officials decreed that the Cancer Control Society could no longer publish the Cancer Control Journal. The reason was that this magazine supplied information to help cancer victims. Did the Society bow to this bureaucratic decree? Of course not! They demanded a hearing in court and won the case. The public health officials were trying to violate the constitutional principles of freedom of the press. The Society had to look like criminals for a while in order to defend the highest law.

Another recent example. The Committee for Freedom of Choice in Cancer Therapy, a nationwide organization based in Los Altos, California, has been fighting for the constitutional rights of cancer victims. They believe that the laws of God and the Constitution of the United States give cancer victims the right to use any harmless food extracts they wish to use.

When supplies of B-17 and other natural substances were seized at the border, the Committee demanded to know on what legal basis such action was taken. The officials were never able to point to any law giving them authority for such seizure. It would have to be assumed then that such seizure had no legal basis and was thus unconstitutional. The Committee continued to demand a legal explanation of these police-state tactics. And no explanation was ever found. But when a savage beast is cornered, he becomes more vicious. The customs official, unable to give any legal explanation for their deeds, reacted by arresting Bob Bradford and Frank Salaman, President and Vice President of the Committee.

This is an age-old technique. When someone proves you wrong in an argument, you can always turn on him personally and destroy him.

These unselfish defenders of our freedom have been indicted by a grand jury, fingerprinted and mugged like common criminals, and required to post bonds higher than those sometimes required of murderers. And for what reason? There is no federal or state law forbidding the alleged actions. There is not even a formal FDA policy prohibiting the import of vitamin B-17. The only document found so far to support this cruelty is an *unsigned* FDA memo stating that Laetrile is an "unapproved new drug." If such a flimsy document is any law at all, it falls at the absolute bottom level of legal authority.

The claim that vitamin B-17 is an "unapproved new drug" is a threefold falsehood. First, it is not a drug, but rather a food. Second, it is not new. The Chinese used it 4000 years ago and it was listed in the U. S. Pharmacopoeia as far back as 1840. Third, it is not unapproved. By common consent, all government agencies approved of this substance for more than a century. No disapproval developed until it was found to be helpful to the cancer patient. How has it become disapproved? By what legal action? Our constitution guarantees that no person may be deprived of anything without due process of law. Since all American citizens formerly had the right to use B-17, by what process of law has this right been removed? There is none. Therefore the claim that B-17 is "disapproved" is false. It cannot become disapproved without due process. Only the FDA could come up with a three word statement containing three falsehoods! "Unapproved new drug," indeed!

I may have some deeply prejudiced reader who cannot be dislodged from his position by all the logic in the world. One may be so blinded by tradition that he may feel that the FDA has the right to ban shipments of B-17. Let's look at an exact parallel and see what you believe. For many years a great many people have been drinking orange juice because they feel that it helps to prevent colds. And the FDA does not interfere. But you can rest assured that if large numbers of people came to believe that orange juice was helpful in case of cancer, the FDA would interfere. They could then ban all shipments of orange juice on the grounds that it was an "unapproved new drug." Those who imported orange juice from Mexico could be imprisoned as criminals. Don't you dare say that this is ridiculous, because it is exactly what has happened to vitamin B-17! There is absolutely no difference in these two situations except one is orange extract and one is apricot extract. If one can be banned as an "unapproved new drug," then so can the other!

Now where do you stand? If you approve of banning apricot extract, but dislike banning orange extract, would you please search your heart for hypocricy? If the reader is an honest American, would you please realize that you have a moral responsibility to fight for the constitution and against unjust, cruel, arbitrary, unreasonable decrees that rob men of freedom and send cancer victims to an early and agaonizing death!

WHEN CHRISTIANS ARE TRICKED INTO FIGHTING AGAINST FREEDOM

The Bible abounds with examples of good men who were deceived into opposing the things of God. The best example is in the case of the public attitude toward Jesus. The scriptures tell us that the common people believed in Him at first because the evidence clearly showed that He was One sent from God. But later they turned against Him. Why? Not because of any change in the evidence, but because of official influence. "Have any of the rulers or of the Pharisees believed on Him?" (John 7:48). This is an age-old problem. Weak men always want to get on the official bandwagon. They want the power and approval that comes from worldly officials. It is part of our natural tendency to compromise with the world. Even Christians are sometimes caught up in this worldly desire to be on the side with the "officials." And it is a dangerous tendency. In our blind desire for official approval we may ignorantly fight against the Lord Himself.

The writer of the letter to the Hebrews warned these professing believers that they were in danger of crucifying the Lord afresh. The context clearly shows what their problem was. They claimed to trust Christ with their souls, but because of their desire to compromise with official policies, they were rebelling against Christ Himself and were in effect denying Him. The same thing can happen to Christians today. When Hitler was committing his horrible atrocities, many professing Christians in Germany went along with him and enjoyed official favor. They were honored as "good citizens." But Martin Niemoller opposed this evil monster and was jailed as a criminal. But now who would you say was criminal and who was a good citizen? Christians must support justice and true law, but we are stupid and cowardly when we are tricked into supporting the fickle and changing decrees of petty men.

Christians can be tricked into supporting evil and they can also be tricked into opposing men of God. For example, Paul was falsely imprisoned, and some of his Christian friends turned against him because of his imprisonment. Why? They had no evidence of wrong doing, but they assumed that the officials could do no wrong and that a man in jail must be a wrong doer. There were other preachers who took advantage of his predicament to poke fun at him (Phil. 1:15-16). No doubt they called him a "jail bird" and pointed to his imprisonment as "proof" of his bad character. Even some of Paul's close friends deserted him because he was in prison. They loved the approval of the world more than they loved the truth. Paul write with sorrow, "Demas hath forsaken me, having loved this present world." How stupid of those ancient people to be guilty of such shallow thinking! Indeed! But Christians today (and some preachers) can be just as stupid. We violate all the principles of Christianity and all the principles of Americanism when we judge a man before we know the facts. Our American system of justice declares that a man is innocent until proven guilty. But in actual practice such is usually not the case. When a person is charged, almost invariably he is assumed to be guilty. Christians are often just as ignorant and unfair at this point as others. We assume that one who has been charged must be guilty. And this is in plain defiance of clearly stated Biblical principles (Prov. 18:13). As an example of such folly I can refer again to the arrest of the officers of the Committee for Freedom of Choice in Cancer Therapy. They have been charged with carrying apricot extract across the border. Big deal! What law forbids it? Nothing but an unsigned FDA memo which is itself clearly contrary to the constitution. Fortunately most honest Americans are intelligent enough to see through such a shallow charge as this, and can see that these men are defending our constitutional freedoms. But no doubt a few simple minded Americans will use the same logic as in the days of Paul and will assume them to be wrongdoers because they have been charged. Truly, history does repeat itself!

We must remember that a man is not guilty until convicted in court. And he still is not guilty until the decision is upheld by the Supreme Court, and the real Supreme Court has not met yet on this issue, for I refer to the Supreme Court of Heaven.

WHICH SIDE WILL YOU BE ON WHEN THIS COURT MEETS?

Christians especially had better be very careful about condemning those who are fighting to defend our freedoms. We had better be careful about believing every lie printed about them in worldly newspapers, for the Lord will not hold us guiltless. If we criticize those who are fighting for freedom of choice, then we may lend strength to those who deprive dying cancer patients the right to the pain relief of vitamin B-17. How about it Christian, are you willing to sit by and watch a man die in horrible agony, his B-17 snatched from his hand by heartless bureaucrats? Are you willing to lend support to the heartless bureaucrats and criticise those who try to send relief to the dying? What will you say when you stand before the Lord?

I never fully understood this serious Christian responsibility of fighting for our freedoms until I became a cancer patient. This is another reason why I can thank God for allowing me to become a cancer victim. The lessons have been valuable. Now I understand the enormous scope of the fight we are in. And I hope you understand too.

NOW WHICH SIDE ARE YOU GOING TO FIGHT FOR, OPPRESSION AND DEATH, OR FREEDOM AND LIFE?

DO YOU PASS BY?

Paraphrased from *Let The Patients Live* by Wynn Earl Westover, The Shepherd's Crooke Press, Box 1770, Sausalito, Ca.

A certain man went down from Jerusalem to Jericho, and becoming ill, stopped to rest by the wayside, where he was set upon by thieves, which stripped him of his raiment and all his worldly goods and departed, leaving him half dead.

And by chance there came down that way a certain FDA official, and when he saw him, he said to himself: "That man is already half dead. He should be cut apart piecemeal with knives, or if that doesn't work, he should be burned into charred pieces, and if the body is still warm, he must then be given poisonous chemicals—and that should fix it."

But in his mind this FDA official excused himself from administering this program because, he said, "Such a prescription should be administered by those qualified to cut piecemeal, burn, and administer poison." And so he passed by on the other side.

And likewise a Customs Official, passing along the road, when he was at that place came and looked on the unfortunate traveler, lying half dead by the wayside. And when he saw him, he said unto himself, "The FDA has prescribed how this traveler's misfortune should be treated; I cannot become involved in helping—not even to bring him a cup of water. My job is to stop unqualified persons from interfering with the FDA's prescription for such luckless travelers." And he too passed by on the other side.

But a certain Samaritan as he journeyed came where the traveler lay, and when he saw him he had compassion on him, and instead of passing by on the other side, went to him and bound up his wounds, pouring in natural healing substances, vitamins, and apricot extracts and other healing balms, set him upon his own beast and brought him to an inn in the next country and took care of him.

And after many days, when he departed, he took out two pence and gave them to the host and said unto him: "Take care of him, and whatsoever thou spendest more, when I come again I will repay thee." And he departed.

And seeing this, the officials consulted their law books to try and find ways to entrap the good Samaritan upon his return from the far land that they might punish him as a warning to all others, Samaritans or not, who, seeing a sick and injured wayfarer lying by the side of the road, might be tempted in that moment to stop and render healing instead of passing by on the other side.

Do you see the millions dying needlessly of cancer? Please don't pass by on the other side! Won't you help them? Won't you tell them there is hope in God's natural methods? Won't you pray for God to deliver them from the cruel American Cancer Monopoly? Won't you please write your congressman and ask him to lift the foolish FDA ban on amygdalin? Or will you too just pass by on the other side?

APPENDIX

The information supplied in this appendix is given in response to many requests. The addresses have been taken from other published sources and are believed to be correct. Such information is of course subject to error and to change. Any errors are regretted, and if discovered will be corrected in future printings.

When writing to any of these organizations for information, be sure to enclose a stamped, self-addressed envelope. If this is not done, heavy mail volume may make reply impossible.

There is a very limited supply of non-toxic cancer therapies. Many clinics are full and may not be able to accept new patients. Always secure an appointment before appearing at any clinic. Persons seeking either orthodox or unorthodox treatments should investigate the doctor, the treatment, and the price before deciding on a course of action. This writer is not in position to recommend or endorse any of the organizations listed in this appendix. The information is given for educational purposes only.

FOR METABOLIC THERAPY AND CONTACTS CONCERNING B-17 THERAPY

The Committee for Freedom of Choice
In Cancer Therapy
146 Main St., Suite 408
Los Altos, CA 94022
Phone (415) 948-9475
They can supply the name of a physician near you.

OTHER NON-TOXIC CANCER THERAPIES

Eva Hill
22 Paterson St.
Hamilton, New Zealand
(Hoxsey Herbal Therapy)

Ivy Cancer Research Foundation
622 W. Diversey Parkway
Chicago, IL 60614
Phone (312) 327-1456
(Carcalon Therapy)

Mrs. Charlotte Strauss
71-40 112th St.
Forest Hills, NY 11375
Phone (212) 263-2190
(Information about Dr. Gerson's nutritional therapy)

FOR NUTRITIONAL PROGRAMMING

Any Physician Belonging To:
The American Academy of Medical Preventics or Contact: HARPER MD.

THE HORMONE TEST FOR CANCER DETECTION

(1) Place one cupful rubbing alcohol in a clean gallon jug.

(2) Collect in this jug all urine passed in a 24-hour period. Keep sample cool, refrigerate in summer, shake occasionally.

(3) At end of 24-hour period, shake again, pour at least 4 ounces of sample into plastic bottle, discard remainder.

(4) Attach label to bottle, giving name and address of patient.

(5) Tighten lid of bottle thoroughly, pack in carton surrounded by crumpled newspapers or other cushion-type packing.

(6) Enclose check or money order for $10.00 in package and send by airmail to any of the following laboratories. (This information and price quotation is furnished by Dr. Contreras, but it is believed that instructions and prices are similar at the other laboratories.)

> Ernesto Contreras, M.D.
> P.O. Box 3793
> San Ysidro, CA 92073
>
> Manuel Navarro, M.D.
> 3553 Sining, Morningside Terrace
> Santa Mesa
> Manila 2803, Philippines

FOR INFORMATION ABOUT METABOLIC SUBSTANCES

These addresses are taken from other published sources, and are reportedly dealers in vitamins and other natural metabolic substances (not drugs). Some do not supply B-17; others may. All conform to legal regulations. Write for catalogs and prices.

A.O. Med. Supply
9498 Lancaster Rd. S.W.
Hebron Ohio 43025
614-928-5161

HAAS Metabolics
P.O. Box 12444
Fort Worth Texas 76108
817-448-8442

Henderson Ph.
7401 Harford Rd.
Baltimore MD. 21234

Libenity Supplies
Castro St.
Mountain View California
415-965-1776

Lemon Metabolics
3030 South Dixie Hwy
West Palm Beach Florida-33405
305-655-2618

Heinsohn Metabolic Supplies
Millet Pit and Seed Co.
RT. #2 Norton Creek Rd.
Gatlinburg Tenn. 37738
615-436-5477

M. Thome
8610 Drawer
Anchorage Alaska 99508
907-279-1082

O. Miller
408 S. Seventh St.
Ord Nebraska 68862
308-728-3251

For information regarding Nation and World Wide Patient Referal contact the Committee for Freedom of Choice in cancer therapy 146 Main St. Suite 408, Los Altos, CA 94022
415-948-9475

RECOMMENDED READING

Prices are approximate and subject to change. Contact

book sources for complete information.

> Publications available from
> AMERICAN OPINION
> BELMONT, MASS. 02178.
>
> *None Dare Call It Conspiracy*, $1.00
> by Gary Allen

A shocking expose of the secret financial powers that control governments from behind the scenes. Explains how government agencies are maneuvered to promote the interests of special groups. This book will make it easy to understand who is keeping Laetrile off the market for their own financial interests.

Vitamins, Federal Bureaucrats Want To Take Yours, 75c
by Gary Allen

Laetrile, Freedom of Choice in Cancer Therapy, 50c
by Alan Stang

Publications available from

THE COMMITTEE FOR FREEDOM OF CHOICE
IN CANCER THERAPY
146 MAIN ST., SUITE 408
LOS ALTOS, CA 94022
PHONE (415) 948-9475.

*the choice
*the inspiring monthly publication about the scientific, political and legal status of laetril. the finest of its kind $10.00 yearly

Anatomy of a Coverup, $3.50
commentary by Dr. Ernst T. Krebs, Jr.

This explosive book presents evidence to indicate that Sloan-Kettering Cancer Research Center has found vitamin B-17 effective on animal cancer, but that the results of the tests have been hidden due to political pressure. If America reads this book, it could turn the country upside down.

Vitamin B-17: Forbidden Weapon Against Cancer, $9.50
by Mike Culbert

A crusading newspaperman exposes the vast medical-legal conspiracy that is keeping Laetrile off the market.

World Without Cancer, 2 volume set, $4.50
by G. Edward Griffin

A highly documented analysis of the Laetrile controversy. One volume presents the scientific background, and the other volume exposes the political and economic conspiracy against Laetrile.

The Laetriles in the Prevention and Control of Cancer, $2.50
by Ernst T. Krebs

A scientific treatise on the chemical behavior of Laetrile, with case histories of successful Laetrile treatment. The reader should have some background in chemistry

Vitamin B-15, $1.25
by V. O. Medexport

A clinical report of successful B-15 treatment in Russia.

A Critical Survey of the State of Cancer, $1.00
by Hans A. Nieper, M.D.

A report of successful cancer treatment using Laetrile, by an outstanding German cancer researcher.

Nutrition Rudiments in Cancer, 75c
by S. M. Jones, M.D.

Basic principles of nutrition for the cancer victim. Also contains much background information on Laetrile.

Amygdalin, The Non-Toxic Analgesic, 75c
(For physicians only)

Explains how amygdalin reduces cancer pain, with testimonies from many world-famous cancer scientists.

The Choice, monthly publication, $10.00 yearly

Up to date news and information about the scientific, political, and legal status of Laetrile.

Also numerous papers-reports pamphlets on the science, politics and therapy of cancer, and other metabolic diseases. Write or phone for complete list, or specific information.

Publications of
The McNaughton Foundation
are available from the
Committee For Freedom of
Choice in Cancer Therapy
146 Main St. Suite 408
Los Altos CA. 94022
Phone 415-948-9475

Technical information for physicians concerning the administration of Laetrile therapy.

The Clergyman's Role in Terminal Cancer, 10c

This pamphlet explains how terminal cancer patients can be delivered from pain and from stupefying drugs by the use of God-given vitamin B-17. This enables the patient to be alert, to make spiritual decisions, and to meet death with dignity rather than as a vegetative narcotics addict. Every clergyman will appreciate this information because of its immensely vital spiritual implications.

THE CANCER CONTROL SOCIETY
2043 Berendo St Los Angeles CA 90027

Numerous Book and pamphlets on cancer, chronic diseases and nutrition-Write for complete list

Publications available from
NATURAL FOODS ASSOCIATES
ATLANTA, TEXAS.

Please Doctor, Do Something! $6.25
by Joe D. Nichols, M.D.

An interesting basic textbook on natural foods and health. Written by an orthodox physician who for years believed the AMA and FDA propaganda line until his own heart attack started him down the road to natural health.

Publications available from
PERSONAL CHRISTIANITY,
BOX 157
BALDWIN PARK, CA 91706

Jesus Wants You Well!, $4.25
by C.S. Lovett, D.D.

A spiritual and practical book with convincing arguments that God desires health for His children. Practical guidance on how to cooperate with the Great Physician.

Death Made Easy, $2.25
by C.S. Lovett, D.D.

A most unusual book which helps to take the fear out of death for the Christian. Gives sensible guidance about preparing for death and making the funeral a testimony for Christ. Definitely not morbid reading, but filled with hope and encouragement.

Index

Acid-alkaline balance, 76
Adam's curse, not responsible for disease, 21
Almonds, in cancer therapy, 79
American diet, controversy over, 25
Amygdalin, see Vitamin B-17
Anti-Christian, to fail to resist unjust law, 260
Atheism, defined, 88-89
Atheistic assumptions of science, 89-90

Balance of nature, 69
Beard, John, discoverer of the true nature of cancer, 61
Beta-glucosidase, 82
Bible, example of good men, 267
Biopsy, in cancer detection, 143
Body, its own healer, 30; programmed for healing, 14; soul and spirit, 252

Bond, posted, 265
Bouziane, N.R., M.D., successful use of B-17, 108
Bradford, Bob, 265
Breast cancer controversy, 92
Bruno, burned at stake for scientific discoveries, 90
Bureaucratic procedure, 255; violates Constitution, 256; petty edict, 262
Bureaucrats, and unconstitutional methods, 118, 135; harassment of B-17, 141, 158, 159-160; methods used to destroy cancer researchers, 121-122
Burk, Dean, cancer researcher, 109, 117, 141

Calcium diorotate, 142
Cancer Control Society, 264
Cancer detection: biopsy, 143; hormone test, 143; X-ray, 142-143

Cancer industry, founded on atheism, 95
Cancer monopoly, 249
Cancer trap, 131
Cancer treatment, in America a failure, 59
Cartier, Jacques, and Vitamin C, 49
Case histories, 128
Chaparral, in cancer therapy, 75
Chemotherapy, as cancer treatment, 132; in nature, 82
Chorionic gonadotropin, 143
Christian responsibility and B-17, 147; responsibility to heal, 252-253; support metabolic therapy, 253-254; attitude toward lw, 256; unselfish defenders of freedom, 265; fighters for freedom, 271
Christianity, 251; God provided healing, 251; responsibility to heal, 252
Christians and the law, 133
Christians in government agencies, responsibility of, 150
Christians in healing professions, responsibility of, 149
Chronic diseases, and failure of American medicine, 34; defined, 26; due to faulty nutrition, 34
Committee for Freedom of Choice in Cancer Therapy, 144; fighting for constitutional rights, 264-270
Conspiracy against B-17, 120
Constitution, and cancer law, 134; showing disrespect, 254; doesn't automatically correct bad law, 263; Health Department violates, 264; contrary to, 270
Contreras, Ernesto, M.D., successful use of B-17, 108; bond posted, 265; criminal, 264; don't brand as, 267-268
Courage, to stand for highest law, 257; Christian needed today, 258
Court, US District, 256
Courts, test law in, 262; Federal courts rule against unconstitutional law, 262

Death, some will escape, 156; what it means for Christians, 157
Dentists, in cancer control, 145
Discrimination against cancer victims, 119
Disease, God not responsible for, 12, 21; man responsible for, 20
Diseases, chronic, and natural foods, 26

Emotions and health, 40
Enzymes, in cancer therapy, 73

Eternal life, how to be sure of, 154
Exercise, and health, 40

Faith, not sufficient basis for all healing, 37
Falsehood used against B-17, 116
Fasting, 79
FDA, opposition to vitamins, 55; memo, 265; falsehood, 266, 270-272
Fiber, importance in the diet, 78
Fold medicine, 71
Food, Bible emphasis on, 16; for body building, 15
Food supply, destroyed by man, 24
Foods containing vitamin B-17, 139
Freedom, 250; political, 250; principles of, 260; pioneers of, 264; unselfish defenders of, 265; support fighters for, 271
Freedom of choice, honest men must support, 249-250

Galileo, imprisoned for scientific discoveries, 90
Gerson, Max, M.D., persecuted for his cancer discoveries, 100
God's cancer treatments, legal opposition to, 98; given methods, 253; natural immunilogical system, 253; will hold us responsible, 256; will punish injustice, 259; laws of, 264
Goldberger, Joseph, M.D., opposed for his conquest of Pellagra, 51
Government, proper role of, 124; branches of, 256; agents suppress needed relief, 259
"Grape Cure" for cancer, 74

Johanna Brandt

Harvey, William, persecuted for his discovery of the circulatory system, 49
Healers, all types are successful, 32
Health, an individual responsibility, 29; damaged by urban life, 27; programmed in nature, 13; natural avenues superior to unnatural, 250; samaritan, 273
Health food stores, 137
Health literature, 138
Heaven, how to get there, 155
Hippocrates, oath of, 135
History of medical profession, 48-53
Hitler, used law to murder, 258; continues, 259-268
Holy Spirit, templed in Christian's body, 14, 31
Hormone test for cancer, 142; instructions, 185
Hoxsey, Harry, persecuted for his cancer discoveries, 100
Hunzas, free from cancer, 85
Hydrazine sulphate, 141

Hypocrisy of forbidding
B-17, 104; submit to unjust
law, 260

Illogical opposition to B-17,
115
Injustice, whether legal or
illegal not acceptable to
God, 257
Inquisition, thousands killed
by law, 258; continues, 259
Ivy, Andrew, persecuted for
his cancer discoveries, 100

Jerusalem to Jericho, a
certain man from, 271
Jesus, commanded to heal,
253; crucified by law, 258;
public attitude toward, 267
Johnson grass, and B-17, 140
Justice, based on nature of
God, 257; good men
concerned with, evil men
manipulate it, 258; lack of,
264

Kell, George, B-17 attorney,
117
Koch, William, M.D.,
persecuted for his cancer
discoveries, 100
Krebs, Ernst, developer of
vitamin B-17, 81

Laetrile, see Vitamin B-17
Law, 254; some law higher
than other, 254; used as
tool of suppression, 256;
God holds us to support
real law, 256; used to
pervert justice, 257; law's
purpose is justice, 257;
officials had none, 265;
due process of, 266;
highest law, 256; bottom
level of law, 265;
higher-lower law, 261;
cannot be classed as
law-breaking, 263;
Nehemiah, 261-264;
violation of, 263; to test
law courageous men must
break law, 263;
responsibility to change
unjust and illegal law, 260
Laws of health, universal, 13
Legal status of vitamin B-17,
135; confusion of, 254;
support of illegal action,
256; legal technicalities;
Gold not interested in, 259;
legality, 260; bureaucratic
opposition, 261
Levels of legal authority, 254,
256
Lord, will not hold us
guiltless, 270, 271

Mankind's self destruction,
23
Medical associations,
interference with medical
progress, 55
Medical doctors, are they
healthy?, 35
Medical organizations, and
unchristian pressure, 36
Medical persecution of other
healers, 54

Medical profession, history of, 48; proper role in health, 29, 34
Medical training in America, 34
Mental attitude and health, 33, 138
Metabolic disease, 127
Metabolic substances, sources, 185
Metabolic therapy, 128, 144, 145; God's natural method, 253; materials for, 140; sources, 184
Metabolism and health, 137
Minerals in cancer therapy, 73
Miracles, emphasis on, sometimes evil, 37; not sufficient basis for all healing, 37
Monopoly in cancer industry, 98, 106, 110, 132, 142
Morrone, John, M.D., successful use of B-17, 107

Natural foods, and cancer therapy, 137; and health of primitive people, 26, defined, 25
Natural healing, sometimes better than supernatural healing, 38
Navarro, Manuel, M.D., successful use of B-17, 107
Nehemiah, 260-261
Nieper, Hans, M.D., successful use of B-17, 107

Non-toxic cancer therapies, 184
Nutrition, faulty, a cause of cancer, 69
Nutritional programming, 185
Nutritional therapy, 145

Official opposition to medical progress, 48-52
Organic gardens, 137

Pancreatic enzymes and cancer, 61, 141
Pangamic acid, 142
Pasteur, Louis, persecuted for his discovery of germs, 51
Paul, apostle, imprisoned illegally, 258; Christians turned against him, 269; days of Paul, 270
Pellagra, official opposition to its cure, 51
Penicillin, officially opposed, 52
Physicians, persecuted for cancer successes, 152
Plant life, the source of health, 17
Plants and healing in the Bible, 18
Pollution and disease, 41
Prayer, not sufficient basis for all healing, 39
Preachers' responsibility and B-17, 149
Preventative medicine, 145
Principles of health, are impersonal, 31, 33

Principles of natural health, 136
Processed foods, 25; and chronic diseases, 26
Processing of foods, a cause of cancer, 82
Professional help for cancer victims, 145
Profits, not by promoters but by orthodoxy, 118
Proteins in cancer therapy, 74

Quackery, falsely charged against doctors using B-17, 106

Radiation, as cancer therapy, 132
Reading, list of recommended titles, 186
Rebellion, against true law, 262; moral responsibility, 267
Religious discrimination and B-17, 123
Rhodenase, 82

Salaman, Frank, 265
Salvation, how to find it, 154; health-natural avenues superior to unnatural, 250
Satan, indirectly responsible for disease, 22; is he behind B-17 opposition?, 112; the prince of this world, 45
Scurvy, and vitamin C, 49
Semmelweis, Ignaz, persecuted for conquering childbed fever, 50
Smoking cancer patients, 138
Supreme Court, 258; of heaven, 259, 270
Surgery as cancer therapy, 132

Takaki, Kanehiro, ridiculed for conquering Beri-Beri, 51
Terminal cancer patients, persecuted by FDA, 148
Terminal condition, advantages of, 153; nothing strange, 152
Trophoblast cells, chemistry of, 143
Trophoblast theory of cancer, 59; evidence for, 62-65

Unapproved new drug, 266-267
Unconstitutional character of B-17 opposition, 118
Unfair opposition to B-17, 115
Urban life, the enemy of health, 27

Vegetarianism, not required in Scripture, 18
Vesalius, Andreas, persecuted for his discoveries in anatomy, 49
Virus theory of cancer, 57-59; compared with trophoblast theory, 66-77
Vitamin B-1, and beri-beri, 51
Vitamin B-2, and pellagra, 56

Vitamin B-15, 142
Vitamin B-17, dishonest basis of legal opposition, 102-103; evidence in favor of, 83-86; false charges against, 106-112; history, 81; non-toxic, 109; therapy, sources, 162; court forbids, 259; Vitamin B-17, 265-266, 271
Vitamin C, and scurvy, 49
Vitamin C, opposed for 260 years, 49
Vitamins in cancer therapy, 73

Washington, George, bled to death by physicians, 50

Who supports Freedom of Choice?, 250
Witch doctor treatments, 94
World, opposed to God's healing, 44; the Bible definition of, 44; under Satan's leadership, 45
World of medicine, often against God, 47, 53
World of religion, often against God, 46, 53

X-ray, in cancer detection, 143

Yogurt, in cancer therapy, 75